HOW TO PARTNER WITH GIRL SCOUT SENIORS ON

SOW WHAT?

IT'S YOUR PLANET—LOVE IT! A LEADERSHIP JOURNEY

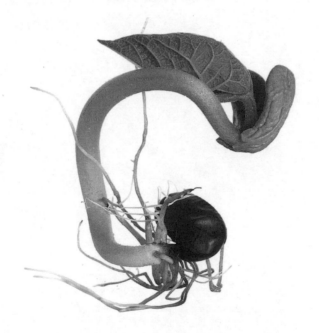

*A Girl Scout leadership journey invites girls to explore a theme
through many experiences and from many perspectives.
All the joys of travel are built right in: meeting new people, exploring new things,
making memories, gathering keepsakes. This guide is your suitcase.
It's packed with everything you need for a wonderful trip that will change girls' lives.*

Girl Scouts of the USA

CHAIR,
NATIONAL BOARD
OF DIRECTORS
Connie L. Lindsey

CHIEF
EXECUTIVE
OFFICER
Kathy Cloninger

VICE
PRESIDENT,
PROGRAM
Eileen Doyle

Girl Scouts

WRITERS: Naomi Person, Valerie Takahama

CONTRIBUTORS: Toi James, Kate Gottlieb,
David Bjerklie, Kathleen Sweeney

DESIGNED BY Alexander Isley Inc.

EXECUTIVE EDITOR, JOURNEYS: Laura Tuchman

MANAGER, OPERATIONS: Sharon Kaplan

GSUSA DESIGN TEAM: Sarah Micklem, Rocco Alberico

© 2009 by Girl Scouts of the USA

First published in 2009 by Girl Scouts of the USA
420 Fifth Avenue, New York, NY 10018-2798
www.girlscouts.org

ISBN: 978-0-88441-741-5

Printed in Italy

1 2 3 4 5 6 7 8 9/17 16 15 14 13 12 11 10 09

Page 16: photo courtesy of Natural Lands Trust.
Page 59: illustration by Suzanne Stryk.
Page 89: illustration by Hadley Hooper.

Text printed on Fredrigoni Cento
40 percent de-inked, post-consumer
fibers and 60 percent secondary
recycled fibers.

Covers printed on Prisma artboard
FSC Certified mixed sources.

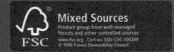

Mixed Sources
Product group from well-managed
forests and other controlled sources
www.fsc.org Cert no. SQS-COC-100209
© 1996 Forest Stewardship Council
FSC

CONTENTS

FOOD FOR THOUGHT 5

    Food Prints and Leader Prints, Too 6

    Toward the Harvest Award 8

    Snapshot of the Journey 10

    Health, Safety, and Well-Being 12

    Digging into Math, Science, and Engineering 14

SENIORS AND THE GREAT OUTDOORS 16

    Girl Scout Ceremonies and Traditions 18

WHAT + HOW: CREATING A QUALITY EXPERIENCE 20

    Seeing Processes Play Out in *Sow What?* 22

    Understanding the Journey's Leadership Benefits 24

    From *GIRLtopia* to *Sow What?* 26

    Your Perspective on Leadership 27

THE JOURNEY'S 10 SAMPLE SESSIONS 29

    What You'll Find in Each Session 30

    Customizing the Journey 31

    Family, Friends, and an Ever-Growing Circle 32

    Session 1: So What About *Sow What?* 34

    Session 2: Foraging for Food 50

    Session 3: What Makes a Meal Really Happy? 54

    Session 4: Dig Deeper 60

    Session 5: *Sow What?*: Global Outlook 64

    Session 6: Planning to Harvest 72

    Session 7 & 8: Harvest Time! 82

    Session 9 & 10: Reap What You Sow! 90

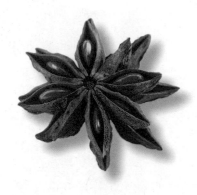

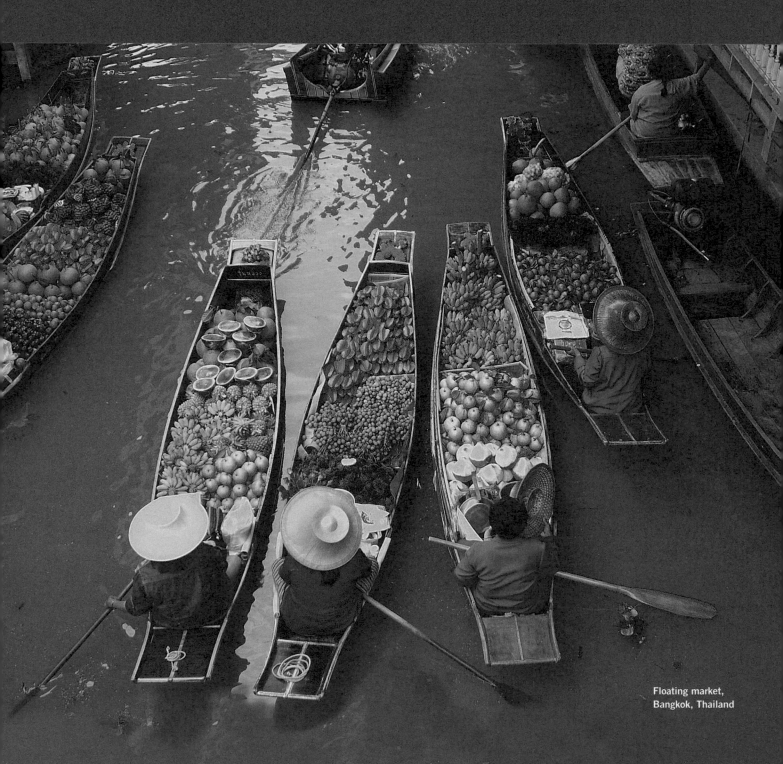

"We're trying to work with nature . . . But we also feel that social issues and community issues are an equally important part of the whole balance."

— Judith Redmond, Full Belly Farm, in the Capay Valley of California

Floating market,
Bangkok, Thailand

Food for Thought

Food is energy. And that energy is part of a vast network that stretches, often for thousands of miles, from the sun and soil through a multitude of people and places before reaching our plates to nourish us.

Food, of course, costs money. With all the conveniences available today, it is all too easy to forget that each and every bite of food also comes at a cost to Earth's resources. So, what and who will protect those resources?

Sow What? invites girls (and you!) on a journey through some big food issues: how and where food is grown, processed, distributed, consumed—and so often wasted. As the girls dig in, they will ask themselves what good they can sow on Earth by adjusting their "food prints" and cultivating sustainable food (and people) networks. When harvest time comes, they will know that a big part of the answer to Sow What? is their own "leader print."

What the girls learn about food networks, and the curiosity that this new knowledge inspires, will be the springboard to caring about our planet now and throughout their lives. The Seniors and you are joining an enduring tradition. Nourishment from the land has been at the core of Girl Scouting since its founding in 1912. "It goes without saying," Girl Scouts founder Juliette Gordon Low once wrote, "that Girl Scouts must have gardens."

The gardens planted on this journey will, for the most part, not be literal ones (although those are possible, too!). The girls may never dig a single shovel into any soil at all (although they might enjoy that!). But everything they do has the same goal as a well-tended garden: a bountiful harvest that continues season after season and year after year. Through Sow What? you have a chance to plant seeds of environmental stewardship that will flourish now and throughout girls' lives. What are you waiting for? Start sowing!

Food Prints and Leader Prints, Too

To engage the Seniors in the global issues food and land use, this journey expands the notion of an environmental footprint into the realm of leadership by having the girls delve into their "food print" *and* their "leader print."

Sow What? also makes use of the word *nourish* in a way that reaches beyond food to relationship issues: Along the journey, girls nourish themselves with a greater understanding of food issues (and actual food!) and they also nourish their personal networks through positive relationship strategies. Making the most of healthy relationship strategies makes girls more effective in teamwork, and in public speaking. That translates into being effective at educating and inspiring others to care about global food networks.

In this way, the journey engages girls in developing into leaders who understand the importance of food networks and why they must be improved, and who can also move forward to make a difference in any arena they choose.

HEARTS AND MINDS

So much information is now available about environmental problems facing our planet and what must be done to correct them. *Sow What?* is part of a series of Girl Scout leadership journeys that invites girls, and their families and adult volunteers, to make sense of that information so they can act for the betterment of Earth.

The umbrella theme for the series—*It's Your Planet—Love It!*—came directly from a brainstorm with teen Girl Scouts. Its sentiment is clear: The desire to nurture and protect is first and foremost an act of love. If girls love Planet Earth and all its wonders—airy and otherwise—they will naturally be moved to protect it. Love for Planet Earth is the true and necessary starting point for thoughtful and sustained environmental action.

YOU'RE ON THIS JOURNEY, TOO!

As you guide girls to Take Action to improve their food networks, you may find yourself adjusting your own food network. If you do, you'll be adding to the harvest the girls reap. And you'll see that when you work to improve food networks across the world, every bite counts!

You may already be deeply committed to environmental causes—or not. Either way, you will be guiding girls on a journey of learning and doing that creates improved food networks in their lives and in the world.

FEEDING SCIENTIFIC MINDS

All along its savory route, *Sow What?* engages girls in science, math, the outdoors, and environmental stewardship. You may be an expert in one or all of these areas—or none. No matter—there's no need to have all the answers! All you need to guide your group of Seniors is right here in this book. Just add your own sense of wonder, and an eagerness to explore all that our food networks offer and accomplish.

Imagine the power of more than 100,000 Seniors and their volunteers and families making choices that improve and protect Earth's food networks. What are you waiting for? Dig in!

SOWING WITH FOCUS

As the Seniors dig into *Sow What?* they'll find a wealth of issues to focus on. If they've journeyed through *GIRLtopia*, encourage them to make use of their already highly developed girl lens— it's a great way to view food networks, too.

Toward the Harvest Award

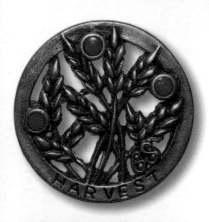

During the *Sow What?* journey, girls have an opportunity to earn the prestigious Girl Scout Senior Harvest Award. The Harvest Award is an important step on the Girl Scout leadership ladder; it signifies that girls understand who they are and what they stand for, and that they care about others, too. It also signifies that they can grasp an issue by the roots and organize a team to work together to sow the seeds of sustainable change.

To earn the Harvest Award, Seniors will complete three steps, which they can accomplish—as a team or on their own. Here are the steps, which are also detailed on pages 86–89 of the girls' book:

1 **Get your leader print going! Here's the path:** Identify, and dig into, a food or land issue, tapping some community experts as you go.

Maybe you've met growers, gardeners, nutritionists or others in your region and have ideas about challenges they face. Maybe you've improved your food print and want to inspire others. Want your school to host a farmers' market? Got a seed of an idea from this book? Want to team up with other Seniors? Just choose an issue that allows you to use your unique talents and learn something new, too!

2 **Capture your vision for change in a Harvest Plan that includes:** Your very own "So What?"—your goal, why it matters, how it will benefit both the planet and people. Say it in a way that gets others interested and involved! Show how even simple actions and decisions impact the larger food network.

Remember: There's no need to go it alone. Who can you turn to for input and support?

What specific impact do you hope to have? Name it! And when you have executed your plan, check back. Have you achieved it? Maybe you will have achieved other results, too, especially if you find yourself needing to adjust your plans along the way.

Your project can be big or small, depending on your time and interest. Either way, strive for a sustainable impact. You may push for a new policy or for a change in an existing one. You don't need to start something from scratch.

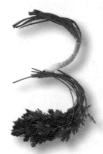 **Now, create change**—execute your plan by advocating to influence a food policy or land-use effort (yes, you can!), or by educating and inspiring others to act on a solution you identify.

As the girls move through the steps toward the Harvest Award, encourage them to take time to stop, think, and reflect along the way. You might say:

- *Do you need to adjust anything based on new information you're learning? Are any new challenges arising?*

- *Be sure to ask adults in your network for success tips! Incorporate the best methods and styles into your own work.*

- *What are you doing that surprises you? Are you speaking up more? Solving a problem you thought you couldn't? Take pride in how you are growing!*

- *Think about your team, too. Are you happy with the way everyone is working together? Is there anything you need to talk about? Courageous conversation, anyone?*

- *Who have you educated and inspired to take action along with you? That matters because getting more people in the know means your impact can have a wide reach!*

A GOOD HARVEST PROJECT PLAN . . . "

- gives the girls the opportunity to expand their network.

- is realistic based on the girls' time and interest.

- uses the Seniors' unique skills and talents.

- helps the girls learn something they can apply to their lives.

- contributes to sustainable change.

- gives them an opportunity to advocate, and to educate and inspire.

CRITICAL THINKING MORE IMPORTANT THAN PROJECT "SIZE"

The amount of time girls spend on their Harvest project is less important than their having a meaningful opportunity to identify, plan, and do the project. If the girls have already enjoyed the *GIRLtopia* leadership journey, revisit the coaching steps spelled out in its Take Action Planning Chart. The learning that takes place along the way is what will benefit girls now and all their lives. The girls might also revisit the simpler version of that chart on page 80 of their *GIRLtopia* book.

Snapshot of the Journey

SESSION 1

So What About *Sow What?*

The Seniors become aware of their place in the global food network as they start to think about where food really comes from and how their choices about food impact Planet Earth. They begin to customize their *Sow What?* journey in order to make a real difference in the food network. The girls also:

- make plans to conduct a community Food Forage

SESSION 2

Foraging for Food!

The Seniors explore the food network in their communities and gather ideas, information, and contacts they can use as they think about how to improve their involvement in the food network. The girls:

- conduct field work to scope out how their community grows, buys, and uses food; what is available to whom; and the costs and convenience
- reflect on lessons about diversity that they draw from their field work
- meet/find anyone who might become part of their Harvest network

SESSION 3

What Makes a Meal Really Happy?

The Seniors explore the pleasures of the "local harvest" as they consider all the "ingredients" that go into experiencing a truly happy meal. They then compare this experience to some of their day-to-day encounters with food and the food network. The girls also:

- think about what makes relationships nourishing, too

SESSION 4

Dig Deeper

The Seniors investigate local agricultural practices and find out what some of the challenges are for people who produce food in their region and for the larger food network. The girls also:

- compare soil samples
- consider a range of options, from learning about food connections in their families to the waste-saving benefits of composting

SESSION 5 *Sow What?*: Global Outlook	The Seniors focus their attention on the global issue of hunger, considering how their own decisions and actions impact the food network around the world. The girls also: • consider the values represented by the various women featured in their books, and how they and these women are connected • share their gratitude for the food and nurturing they have in their lives
SESSION 6 Planning to Harvest	The Seniors identify their project for the Harvest Award. The girls: • check in on their commitments, and their teamwork and healthy relations • consider the importance of advocacy in their project
SESSION 7 & 8 Harvest Time!	The Seniors team up and carry out their efforts to have a positive impact on the food network, en route to earning their Harvest Awards. The girls: • consider career opportunities highlighted by the journey • consider the pros and cons of life's "monocultures" • assess healthy relationships • create a food ceremony or festival
SESSION 9 & 10 Reap What You Sow!	The Seniors conclude their *Sow What?* journey, assessing what they have learned, connecting with all those who have assisted them, and celebrating their Harvest. The girls also: • share their Harvest projects with others and see if any ideas emerge about keeping the effort going • consider a range of celebratory options, including stories of growing, sowing, and sewing

Health, Safety, and Well-Being

The emotional and physical safety and well-being of girls is of paramount importance in Girl Scouting. Look out for the safety of girls by following *Safety-Wise* when planning all gatherings and trips, and:

- check into any additional safety guidelines your Girl Scout council might provide, based on local issues
- talk to girls and their families about special needs or concerns

Welcoming Girls with Disabilities

Girl Scouting embraces girls with many different needs and is guided by a very specific and positive philosophy of inclusion that benefits all: Each girl is an equal and valued member of a group with typically developing peers.

As an adult volunteer, you have the chance to improve the way society views girls with disabilities. One way to start is with language. Your words have a huge impact on the process of inclusion. People-First Language puts the person before the disability:

SAY	INSTEAD OF
She has autism.	She's autistic.
She has an intellectual disability.	She's mentally retarded.
She has a learning disability.	The girl is learning-disabled.
She uses a wheelchair.	She is wheelchair-bound.
She has a disability.	She is handicapped.

LEARN WHAT A GIRL NEEDS

First, don't assume that because a person has a disability, she needs assistance or special accommodations. Probably the most important thing you can do is to ask the individual girl or her parents or guardians what she needs to make her experience in Girl Scouts successful. If you are frank with the girl and her parents and make yourself accessible to them, it's likely they will respond in kind, creating a better experience for all.

It's important for all girls to be rewarded based on their best efforts—not on completion of a task. Give any girl the opportunity to do her best and she will. Sometimes that means changing a few rules or approaching an activity in a more creative way. Here are a few examples:

- Invite a girl to perform an activity after observing others doing it first.

- Ask the girls to come up with ideas on how to adapt an activity.

- Often what counts most is staying flexible and varying your approach. For a list of resources, visit www.girlscouts.org and search on "disability resources."

GIRL SCOUT COUNCIL CONTACT INFO

Name: _____

_____

_____

Can help with: _____

_____

_____

Phone: _____

E-mail: _____

Digging into Math, Science, and Engineering

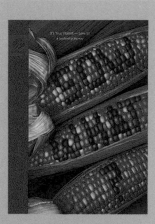

GUIDE THE SENIORS TO SEEK OUT ROLE MODELS

Use the women featured in the girls' book as inspiration to find local role models for the Seniors. Tap your own experience and enthusiasm, and the resources of other women in your community. In the process, you will expand your own horizons— and your appreciation of how science, technology, engineering, and math can be used to make a difference in the world.

*S*ow What? directly engage girls in understanding the scientific fact that life on Earth depends on food. People, animals, plants, microscopic organisms—everything alive needs nourishment.

As the Seniors learn about the food networks all around them, they will see that science, math, and engineering are as much a part of daily life as the food they eat. Yet a troublesome gap often develops between girls' interest and ability in these subjects and their desire and confidence to pursue higher education, and ultimately careers, in these fields. By eighth grade, only half as many girls as boys in the United States are interested in careers in science, technology, engineering, and math (STEM). Those numbers get even worse in high school and college. Fewer than 1 in 5 of all college engineering degrees are awarded to women. And even among these women, a great many leave the profession in their 30s and 40s. Women are also under-represented in the fields of chemistry and physics.

BUILDING SCIENTIFIC MINDS

To sustain interest and build confidence, Girl Scouts believes that exposure to the joys and wonders of these subjects is crucial—as is encouragement from families, teachers, and the media that is so much a part of daily life. What's key is ending the many myths and biases that girls encounter when pursuing these subjects. The other part of the challenge is for girls to realize that science, technology, engineering, and math offer ways to help people and communities. On this journey, Seniors have a direct opportunity to experience how essential these subjects are to any desire to protect Planet Earth. This journey aims to foster lifelong interests in those subjects, and in every aspect of food.

So take advantage of each time STEM subjects pop up in the girls' lives. Calculating the water needed by plants and animals on a farm? A lesson in mathematics. Computer-monitored fish-farm tanks? Technology on the farm. Worms wiggling in a fresh compost heap or new shoots pushing up through bare earth? A reminder that nearly everywhere, Earth is teeming with life.

As *Sow What?* makes clear, even time spent in the kitchen involves endless math problems. Cooking combines chemistry and a lot of math—ratios, measurements, proportions. What's a measuring cup, after all, but a basic math tool? A flattened cake pulled from the oven might signal a scientific misfire. Not enough eggs, perhaps? Or no baking powder? And think of breads, cakes, and cookies, and all their exacting needs. Cooks might dispense with measuring tools, but bakers rarely can. Even the most intuitive of them play by the numbers.

Make the most of every creative scientific moment that arises. If you and the girls try your hand at preparing a meal from all local foods, that's a big win for your food mileage, and your food print. Take a bite and prepare to enjoy some savory moments with the girls.

WOMEN IN SPACE

On Oct. 25, 2007, some 200 miles above Earth, the Space Shuttle *Discovery* docked with the International Space Station, the hatches between the ships opened, and the two commanders followed standard NASA etiquette: They shook hands. But this handshake was one for the history books. The commanders of both missions were women: Pam Melroy and Peggy Whitson.

"It was no publicity stunt," says shuttle commander Melroy. Enough women had worked their way into leadership positions at NASA that a handshake like this was now possible.

Many more women work on the ground at NASA. Melroy recalls the women working on just one mission being called together for a photo. "Everyone was amazed and inspired when they realized the room was filled to nearly bursting!" she says.

"The first woman to walk on Mars is in school today. Let's not let her down— let's help her get there."
—Pam Melroy, commander Space Shuttle *Discovery*

15

Seniors and the Great Outdoors

Strolls through farmland, hikes up a mountain in search of wild blueberries, pauses to watch a robin feed her young—all of these firsthand outdoor experiences help lay a foundation for a lasting appreciation of nature. With its food- and land-based themes, *Sow What?* naturally leads girls to see themselves as part of a larger network—a global one that encompasses all of Planet Earth.

So encourage your team of Seniors to get out and explore as much as they can. Hikes, weekend camping trips, kayaking, canoeing—wherever they go, the girls will see food networks all around them. At times, they might see nature's networks encroaching on human ones. Just think of pigeons and squirrels aggressively snatching crumbs from picnickers in city parks. It's often the other way around, too: Humans encroach on the natural foraging grounds of animals.

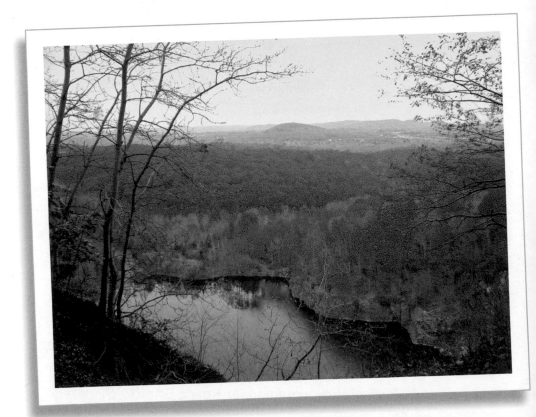

Do mushroom hunters and pickers of wild berries strip the natural feeding grounds that wildlife depends on? When bears eat human food, are they getting needed nourishment or getting out of balance? Is this mingling of human and wild networks good or bad? Or maybe it's not always one thing?

Focusing in on questions like these can help the girls see their place in the world's food networks more clearly. They might even find a way to relate their own human interactions to those they witness in nature. What might they learn about birds in flight or a mother deer protecting her young that they can translate into their own human relationships?

Wherever the girls go, be sure to get them thinking about their food network and how they might reduce their food mileage and their food print. Packing low-mileage snacks is one obvious way to go. What's local and packable for a day hike or overnight camping? What local fruits might make the best snack on a kayaking trip? The Seniors, and you, are sure to have plenty of ideas.

You might even suggest a hike on which the conversation focuses on the top 10 ways to reduce food miles. Invite other girls in the region who are also journeying on *Sow What?* That will ensure more voices, and more ideas, in the mix.

SOLAR CUISINE

Girl Scouts have experimented with solar cooking for decades, and your group might want to try cooking a dish or an entire meal using the sun's powers. Hearty and satisfying three-bean soup, chili pie, zucchini loaf, and even brownie pudding can be made on a solar cooker.

An added plus: Once the food is in the cooker, the girls are free for other adventures.

Girl Scout Ceremonies and Traditions

Even the briefest of ceremonies can take girls away from the everyday to think about hopes, intentions, commitments, and feelings. A ceremony marks a separation from whatever girls have just come from (school, work, dance class, math club) and creates the sense that what will happen now is special and important. So, find out how and when girls want ceremonies.

Girl Scout ceremonies can be as simple as gathering in a circle, lighting a candle, and sharing one hope—or reflecting together on one line of the Girl Scout Law. Or girls might read poems, play music, or sing songs. Invite them to create their own ways to mark their time together as special.

Sharing food, recipes, and meals is a long-standing tradition in Girl Scouts. Along this journey there are many opportunities to continue it. The girls might even do it at every session. They might enjoy these traditions, too:

Quiet Sign

The Quiet Sign is a way to silence a crowd without shouting at anyone. The sign is made by holding up the right hand with all five fingers extended. It refers to the original Fifth Law of Girl Scouting: A Girl Scout is courteous.

SWAPS

Trading SWAPS ("Special Whatchamacallits Affectionately Pinned Somewhere") is a Girl Scout tradition for exchanging small keepsakes. It started long ago when Girl Scouts and Girl Guides from England first gathered for fun, song, and making new friends. Swaps are still a fun way to meet and promote friendship. Each swap offers a memory of a special event or a particular girl—it usually says something about a Girl Scout's group or highlights something special about where she lives. And it's simple; it could be made from donated or recycled goods.

CRAFTY TIP

On this journey, SWAPS can be food- and land-oriented. For example, a girl interested in improving her food miles could make a SWAP representing local foods.

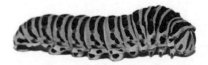

18

Travel

Travel, whether national or local, is a big part of Girl Scouting. Encourage the girls to check out the *destinations* program of travel opportunities at girlscouts.org. For international travel, the World Association of Girl Guides and Girl Scouts (WAGGGS) offers a wealth of opportunities. This umbrella organization for our worldwide sisterhood, founded in 1928, advocates globally on issues of importance to girls and young women. For WAGGGS, as for GSUSA, advocacy means "speaking, doing, and educating." Visits to the four World Centers operated by WAGGGS are highly popular international travel destinations for Girl Scouts. The girls can learn more by searching on "world centers" at girlscouts.org.

Girl Scout Gold Award

Earning the Girl Scout Gold Award is an important tradition in Girl Scouting—and a great way to demonstrate leadership. While on leadership journeys (like this one), girls learn to use the three keys to leadership: Discover, Connect, and Take Action. Then they can go on to earn their Girl Scout Gold Award. Encourage girls to read about the award and girls who have earned it at girlscouts.org. They might ask their council to put them in touch with some of the young women who have earned it before them, so they can receive advice firsthand.

What + How: Creating a Quality Experience

It's not just what girls do, but how you engage them that creates a high-quality Girl Scout experience. All Girl Scout activities are built on three processes that make Girl Scouting unique from school and other extracurricular activities. When used together, these processes—Girl Led, Cooperative Learning, and Learning by Doing (also known as Experiential Learning)—ensure the quality and promote the fun and friendship so integral to Girl Scouting. Take some time to understand these processes and how to use them with Girl Scout Seniors.

Girl Led

"Girl led" is just what it sounds like—girls play an active part in figuring out the what, where, when, how, and why of their activities. So encourage them to lead the planning, decision-making, learning, and fun as much as possible. This ensures that girls are engaged in their learning and experience leadership opportunities as they prepare to become active participants in their local and global communities. With Seniors, you could:

- guide and act as a resource for girls as they plan complex projects
- encourage girls to question or investigate things that they normally take for granted
- encourage girls to take what excites them along the journey and share it with younger girls, peers, and family in a way that allows them to educate and inspire

Learning by Doing

Learning by Doing is a hands-on learning process that engages girls in continuous cycles of action and reflection that result in deeper understanding of concepts and mastery of practical skills. As they participate in meaningful activities and then reflect on them, girls get to explore their own questions, discover answers, gain new skills, and share ideas and observations with others. Throughout the process, it's important for girls to be able to connect their experiences to their lives and apply what they have learned to their future experiences. With Seniors, you could:

KEEP IT GIRL LED

Remember: You want the girls to take a major role in planning and executing this leadership experience. They may first want you to come up with the ideas and plans. *But hold your ground!* This is the girls' experience, and they're up to the challenge.

From beginning to end, keep your eye on what the girls want to do and the direction they seem to be taking. It's the approach begun by Juliette Gordon Low: When she and her associates couldn't decide on a new direction, she often said, "Let's ask the girls!" At each session, ask the girls for any last thoughts on what they've done or discussed.

- act as a resource for girls while they plan hands-on learning experiences for themselves and others

- expose girls to multiple perspectives and resources for problem-solving and designing projects

- encourage documentation of the girls' learning, reflection, and planning for future action, such as creating how-to guides

Cooperative Learning

Through cooperative learning, girls work together toward shared goals in an atmosphere of respect and collaboration that encourages the sharing of skills, knowledge, and learning. Moreover, given that many girls desire to connect with others, cooperative learning may be a particularly meaningful and enjoyable way to engage girls in learning. Working together in all-girl environments also encourages girls to feel powerful and emotionally and physically safe, and it allows them to experience a sense of belonging even in the most diverse groups. With Seniors, you could:

- promote girls' participation in projects that the entire group can work on, and whose scope reaches beyond their familiar communities

- when asked, give guidance so girls can see the connection between individual action and global solutions

- expose girls to multiple ways of learning together, such as through community leaders, research, seminars, films, and videos

LEARNING BY DOING

The girls have many opportunities to reflect on their journey experiences and apply them to their lives throughout *Sow What?* Check out the Attitudes of Gratitude ceremony suggested for Session 1 (page 41). It gives girls a way to reflect on the important role each food network "player" has in their lives.

SAVORING TEAMWORK

Girls will also benefit from speaking openly and often about how their teamwork is going and how they use relationship strategies purposefully to achieve the best results in teamwork and in life. In Session 3, for example, the girls consider "Healthy Relationships at the Table and in Life." While they prepare a meal and then eat it together, they talk with one another about how much more enjoyable it is to share food among people who have healthy relationships—and what exactly a healthy relationship is.

Seeing Girl Scout Processes Play Out in *Sow What?*

irl Scout processes play out in a variety of ways during team gatherings, but often they are so seamless you might not notice them. For example, in Session 1, the Seniors take part in a food network exercise (pages 35–36) that gets them thinking about how their food choices impact the planet. The call-outs below show how the Girl Scout processes make this a learning and growing experience for girls—and up the fun, too! Throughout *Sow What?*, you'll see processes and outcomes play out again and again. Before you know it, you'll be using these valuable aspects of Girl Scouting in whatever Seniors do—from going for the Girl Scout Silver Award to taking a trip to Girl Scout Cookie Activities!

FROM SAMPLE SESSION 1

The Real Food Network

Now it's time for the girls to begin to envision all the resources—Earth's resources and people resources—as well as all the various decisions about those resources, that bring food to their tables. Invite girls to explore where their favorites they've named "come from" (besides the store!).

Start by asking: How many people, animals, and resources of Earth—the sun, water, and air—go into getting our food to us?

Ask the girls to choose a favorite food they've talked about today (or one ingredient in a food) and then tell the story of the web of interactions that brings that food to their table. They can make educated guesses or simply use their imaginations. But they must tell a whole story. You might say:

> Start with what the sun did for it or what water did for it and move forward through all the steps that let this food reach its final destination—you!

AMP IT UP

Depending on the mood and energy of the girls and time available, they might like to add humor or drama by turning this into a guessing game or even a "mini-commercial" about their good favorites. If the team wants to get creative, they might enjoy spending a few minutes preparing their "performance."

This is **Girl Led** with pizzazz! Besides taking the lead in presenting their ideas, they get to put a creative spin on it, making it informative and entertaining!

As the girls think about the world's resources, how people get them, and who gets to use them, they build toward the **Discover outcome, Girls develop critical thinking.** They also begin to gain a greater understanding of how these decisions and policies affect people's lives. This is a key element of the Senior level **Take Action outcome, Girls advocate for themselves and others locally and globally.**

Girls working together to figure out the path food takes to get to them is a good example of **Cooperative Learning**. This activity also has girls making the connection between "local" (their communities) and "global." This is most closely aligned with the **Connect outcome, Girls feel connected to their communities locally and globally.**

The girls might like to do this individually, in mini-teams, or as a large team. They can keep their examples simple—and have some fun, creatively capturing the story/web on a piece of paper or two. To get their stories going, ask them to consider questions like these, that get them thinking through the a full "food time line":

Say your favorite food is an orange. Who planted the seed that became the orange tree? Who decided what kind of seed to plant and how? Where? Maybe in Florida? Who tended the tree? Was it treated with pesticides? Fertilizers? Artificial or natural? Who decided? Where did that stuff come from? When the tree produced fruit, who picked it? Who tasted it? Packed it? Shipped it? Who unloaded it at the store? Priced it? Displayed it for you? Who bought it? How does it taste?

Invite each girl or team of girls to share her/their food network story. Then, guide a short discussion:

- How does our food connect us to Earth?

- How does our food connect us to people?

- When you bite into a piece of food, do you ever think about the people who produce it, pick it, or deliver it to you? Do you ever wonder whether they actually eat this food themselves?

- What are some of the decisions that get made along our food networks? How do they impact people and the planet?

- What ideas are we starting to have about how decisions along our food networks impact health—the health of the environment and our own?

Encourage the girls to research, before the next gathering, more facts on their own to learn how close to the truth their network stories really come. Did they leave out any links in the web? Did they leave out any key people?

These guiding questions lead girls to the **Discover outcome, Girls develop positive values.** They ask girls to go beyond technical or scientific explanations to think about the social and political aspects of food. As they grapple with the answers, the girls may "strengthen their own and others' commitment to being socially, politically and environmentally engaged citizens" in their communities, locally and globally.

This question focuses on the **Discover outcome, Girls gain practical life skills— girls practice healthy living.** It asks girls to consider healthy living as it pertains to their own lives and the environment. It also asks them to think about food in a global context, and from a social and cultural perspective. This is an important and challenging aspect of this outcome for Seniors—"girls show cultural sensitivity in their efforts to promote healthy living in their communities."

This encouragement is part of the adult-girl partnership in the **Girl Led** process. The adult volunteer encourages the girls to confirm or rethink their thoughts through research. This supports the girls in building toward the **Discover outcome, Girls seek challenges in the world**.

Understanding the Journey's Leadership Benefits

Filled with fun and friendship, *Sow What?* is designed to develop the skills and values girls need to be leaders now and as they grow. The journey's activities are designed to enable Seniors to strive toward achieving 11 of 15 national outcomes, or benefits, of the Girl Scout Leadership Experience, as summarized on the next page. Each girl is different, so don't expect them all to exhibit the same signs to indicate what they are learning along the journey. What matters is that you are guiding them toward leadership skills and qualities they can use right now—and all their lives.

For full definitions of the outcomes and the signs that Girl Scout Seniors are achieving them, see *Transforming Leadership: Focusing on Outcomes of the New Girl Scout Leadership Experience* (GSUSA, 2008). Keep in mind that the intended benefits to girls are the cumulative result of traveling through an entire journey—and everything else girls experience in Girl Scouting.

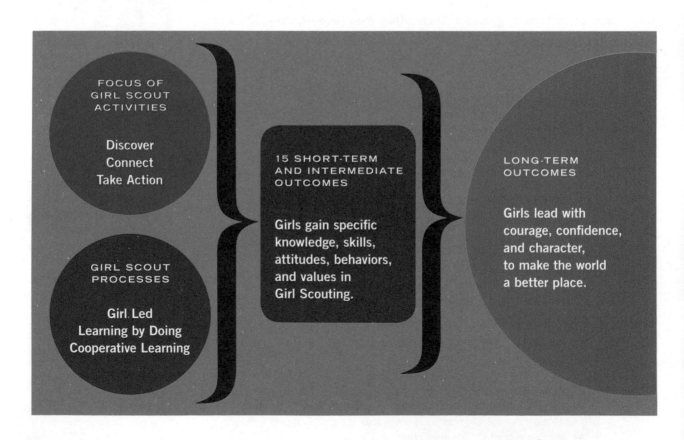

NATIONAL LEADERSHIP OUTCOMES

	AT THE SENIOR LEVEL, girls...	RELATED ACTIVITIES (by Session number or girls' book part/page)	SAMPLE "SIGN" When the outcome is achieved, girls might...
DISCOVER — Girls develop a strong sense of self.	are better able to recognize the multiple demands and expectations of others while establishing their own individuality.	S7 & 8: Career Possibilities	describe challenges they face in finding a balance between accepting group beliefs and thinking/making decisions for themselves.
Girls develop positive values.	strengthen their own and others' commitment to being socially, politically, and environmentally engaged citizens of their communities.	S3: So What Can You Commit To?; GB: Count Your Kernels, p. 45; Your Own BioBlitz, p. 49; So, What About Values?, p. 85	report increased positive attitudes of social responsibility and citizenship.
Girls gain practical life skills—girls practice healthy living.	show cultural sensitivity in their efforts to promote healthy living in their communities.	S1: The Real Food Network; S2: Food Forage; S3: Hunger Pains; S7–S8: Harvest project	report increased knowledge of specific health needs in their diverse communities.
Girls seek challenges in the world.	demonstrate increased enthusiasm for learning new skills and ideas and expanding existing ones.	S2: Food Forage; S3: Agricultural Visit; Harvest Project	increasingly offer their own ideas for exploring new topics or making existing ones more challenging.
Girls develop critical thinking.	are better able to analyze their own and others' thinking processes.	S1: The Real Food Network; S5: Hunger Pain;	give examples of the steps they followed and why they made a specific decision or formed an opinion.
CONNECT — Girls develop healthy relationships.	are better able to recognize and address challenges to forming and maintaining healthy relationships with others	S2, S3, S7 & 8	identify behaviors that hinder the development of positive relationships (e.g., backstabbing, gossip).
Girls promote cooperation and team building.	strengthen their abilities to build effective teams to accomplish shared goals.	S7 & 8: Harvest Project Checklist	identify specific strategies for building effective teams (e.g., paying attention to interests, strengths, team dynamics).
Girls feel connected to their communities, locally and globally.	feel that their connections with diverse members of their communities are important resources for personal and leadership development.	S5: Shared Values, Hunger Pain; GB: All profiles of women and girls	make friends with girls/women through the World Association of Girl Guides and Girl Scouts and can explain why these connections are important to them.
TAKE ACTION — Girls can identify community needs.	are more skilled in identifying their local or global communities' needs that they can realistically address.	S2: Food Forage; GB: Harvest Award Topics, pp. 89–92	report considering multiple factors before deciding on the appropriateness of a project for their community.
		S7 & 8: Who Can You Meet?, Power of More; GB: Cultivate Network, p. 88	seek advice from community members/leaders before selecting issues for action.
Girls advocate for themselves and others.	have a greater understanding of how the decisions and policies of various institutions have effects on their lives and the lives of others.	S9 & 10: Harvest Project Award; GB: Harvest Project, pp. 86–95	report increased knowledge about how public decisions in their schools, communities, and local governments affect people's private lives.
	use advocacy skills and knowledge to be more active on behalf of a cause, issue, or person, locally or globally.		give examples of advocating for an issue in their school or neighborhood.
Girls educate and inspire others to act.	are better at inspiring and mobilizing others to become more engaged in community service and action.	Harvest Project; S10: Harvest Time: Leader Prints; GB: Make It Official, p. 87	shape messages (e.g., in a flier, speech, publication, or Web campaign) to explain the importance of taking action on an issue they care about.
Girls feel empowered to make a difference.	feel that they have greater access to community resources and more equal relationships with adults in their communities.	S9 & 10: Harvest Project Award; GB: Harvest Project, pp. 86–95	report that adults in their communities invite their input and/ or participation in community affairs.

S=Session, GB=Girls' Book

From *GIRLtopia* to *Sow What?*

DON'T GIVE AWAY THE IDEALISM OF GIRLTOPIA!

If *Sow What?* is the first Girl Scout leadership journey your Senior team is embarking on, skip these tips. You wouldn't want to spoil the fun and friendship awaiting the girls on *GIRLtopia* before they have a chance to enjoy it from start to finish! Just go ahead and enjoy *Sow What?*

If your Senior Team has already enjoyed *GIRLtopia*, keep those experiences growing by linking some of its "key" leadership ideas to the *Sow What?* journey. For example, you might ask the girls:

- how do they rate their team dynamic at various points in the journey. Is it higher? Lower? What might they want to improve or change?

- how can their Harvest project let them continue on as visionaries—for the world's food network?

- how can their planned Harvest project better the world for girls?

As the Seniors travel through *Sow What?* take a moment from time to time to get them talking about whether they can take any of the creative energy and ideas, or the creative mediums, of *GIRLtopia* and put them into play during *Sow What?*

And if the Seniors enjoyed taking the lead with "Guide-Its" throughout *GIRLtopia*, by all means continue this new "tradition" in *Sow What?*

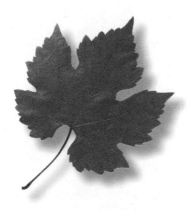

Your Perspective on Leadership

The Girl Scout Leadership philosophy—Discover + Connect + Take Action—implies that leadership happens from the inside out. Your thoughts, enthusiasm, and approach will influence the Seniors, so take some time to reflect on your own perspective on leadership. Take a few minutes now—and throughout *Sow What?*—to apply the three "keys" of leadership to yourself.

Discover	+	Connect	+	Take Action	=	Leadership

DISCOVER What values do you hold related to caring for the environment? Is it ever hard to act on them? Why? What does the Girl Scout Law line "use resources wisely" mean to you?

_____

_____

_____

CONNECT Who would you like to add to your community network? Why do you think it's important for Seniors to connect with an expanding network of people?

_____

_____

_____

TAKE ACTION How does your role as a volunteer with Girl Scout Seniors contribute to making the world—and specifically the environment—better?

_____

_____

_____

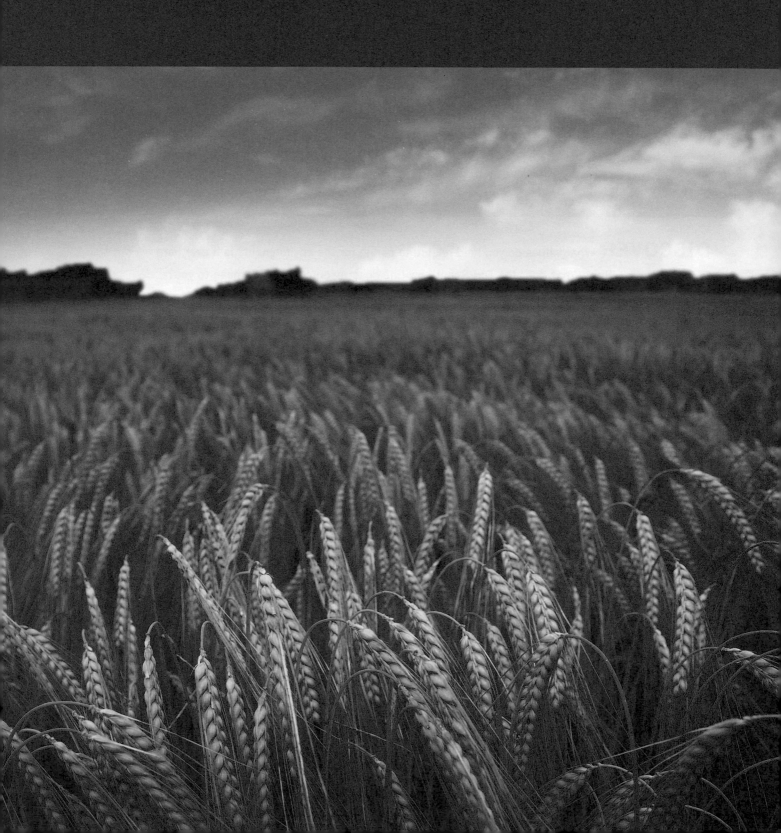

"If you **start with something small**, you can always make it bigger."

— Ivy Vance, Girl Scout from North Liberty, Iowa, who worked to restore a patch of prairie

The Journey's 10 Sample Sessions

As the *Sow What?* journey begins, you'll find it useful to take a little time out to read through the girls' book. Get cozy in your favorite chair, enjoy a favorite food, and dig in!

You'll find that *Sow What?* provides girls with a wealth of interesting ideas about the food network around the world, the leaders at work in it to create more sustainable solutions, possible projects for earning the Harvest award, and some tasty recipes, too! Enjoy it—and encourage girls to enjoy it, too. It's more than a "workbook" for your gatherings. It's a collection of information and inspiration—a springboard for the live experiences you'll have with girls using your guide.

Don't worry about how the girl's book fits into the sessions plotted here for the journey! All the notes and pages to reference are built right into the sample sessions in this section. As you journey with girls, just by following along, you'll be guiding them toward the Harvest Award—and realizing Girl Scouting's leadership benefits! Everything's "sewn in"—from taking time out to talk with girls about healthy relationships (they nourish us, too), to ideas for opening and closing ceremonies to make your gatherings special. Of course, these sessions are only "samples"; you'll tailor them as you go, with the girls—even that's built into the first session's suggestions!

What You'll Find in Each Session

AT A GLANCE: The session's goal, activities, and a list of simple materials you'll need.

What to Say: Examples of what to say and ask the Seniors along *Sow What?* as you link activities, reflections, and learning experiences. Must you read from the "script"? Absolutely not! The girls (and you) will have far more fun if you take the main ideas from the examples provided and then just be yourself.

Activity Instructions: Tips for guiding the girls through activities and experiences along *Sow What?* and plenty of "tools" (lists, charts, suggestions for reflections, etc.) to correspond to the experiences on the journey.

Coaching to Create a Quality Experience: The quality of the Girl Scout Leadership Experience depends greatly on three processes—Girl Led, Learning by Doing, and Cooperative Learning. By following the prompts in this guide for activities, reflections, girl choice-making, and discussions, you'll be using the processes—with ease.

Tying Activities to Impact: This guide notes the purpose of the journey's activities and discussions, so you'll always understand the intended benefit to girls. You'll even be able to see the benefits—by observing the "signs" that the girls are achieving the national Girl Scout Leadership Outcomes.

Customizing the Journey

Part of Sample Session 1 is devoted to giving girls time to shape the journey and its schedule with you, using the "Sow What: Make It Your Own" pages (42–43 in this guide). As you partner with the Seniors, be sure to encourage them to brainstorm some "side trips" that will inspire them to truly make the most of what they can harvest as leaders. Consider for example:

- **Field trips:** Visits to regional sites and organizations related to the topics girls choose for their Harvest projects. These might include farmers' markets, supermarkets, restaurants, gardens, and farms. As resources permit, don't forget to include some time to check out what surrounds these food places or the best place to sample new foods.

- **Networking:** Expand the girls' worldview by partnering with them to identify, and then visit with, adults and college students who can spark their imaginations. During Sessions 7 & 8, for example, when the girls consider career possibilities, perhaps invite women who are flourishing in various food and land-use related careers. The girls can take the lead role in sending invitations and confirming meeting arrangements and other details.

- **Healthy Relationships:** If this interests the girls, find out about ways to tap a community expert or two to offer girls more information about smart strategies for healthy relationships and good communication. If any of the Seniors enjoyed the *aMAZE* Cadette journey last year, which focuses on the twists and turns of getting along, they'll likely want to learn more! So help them find some opportunities to do so.

- **Making Stuff:** Girls who like to make things—crafts, foods, inventions, videos, and other do-it-yourself projects—will enjoy sharing their talents with the team. Those who are good with fabric and thread will appreciate (and may want to take the lead on) the "Sew What" activity suggested in the "Seeds of Fun" section of the Harvest Time! pages (91–92 in this guide), which inspires girls to tell a story with fabric scraps. Encourage all the girls to share their favorite DIYs with one another—perhaps they can even give one another what they make.

PARTNERING WITH GIRL SCOUT SENIORS

Girls in high school are juggling many demands—friendships, grades, sports, drama, dance, music, and other extracurricular activities. Many teens also have the added responsibilities of part-time jobs and/or helping out at home. And, of course, they are always craving opportunities to have fun and just hang out in a space where they feel accepted.

As a volunteer partnering with these busy and sometimes stressed-out girls, you'll want to find just the right balance between providing some much-needed structure and sitting back so that girls explore their own Sow Whats in a way that reflects their needs and interests. This guide offers a range of tips to aid in finding that balance.

Family, Friends, and an Ever-Growing Circle

As the girls plan opening or closing events, ask if they want to invite their families and friends. It's a good way to share the ideas, and perhaps the food, of this bountiful journey.

Girl Scout Seniors will likely have all kinds of ideas for their *Sow What?* journey, and they'll probably want some assistance in carrying them through. Just keep in mind that you don't have to be their only partner. Invite the girls' families and friends to get involved. And encourage the girls to think about other people they can tap. Mobilizing others is a valuable leadership skill.

The girls may even want to reach across the region to other Girl Scout Seniors journeying on *Sow What?* Girls from rural areas might like to see what their urban or suburban peers are doing, and suburban girls might like to see what their urban and rural peers are up to. And when girls from various racial, ethnic, and socioeconomic groups can share ideas, even if just online, they all benefit. They're likely to think even bigger about their food networks. Imagine the power of girls from an entire region sharing their Harvest projects and their ideas for lowering their food prints.

Families and friends	Contact info

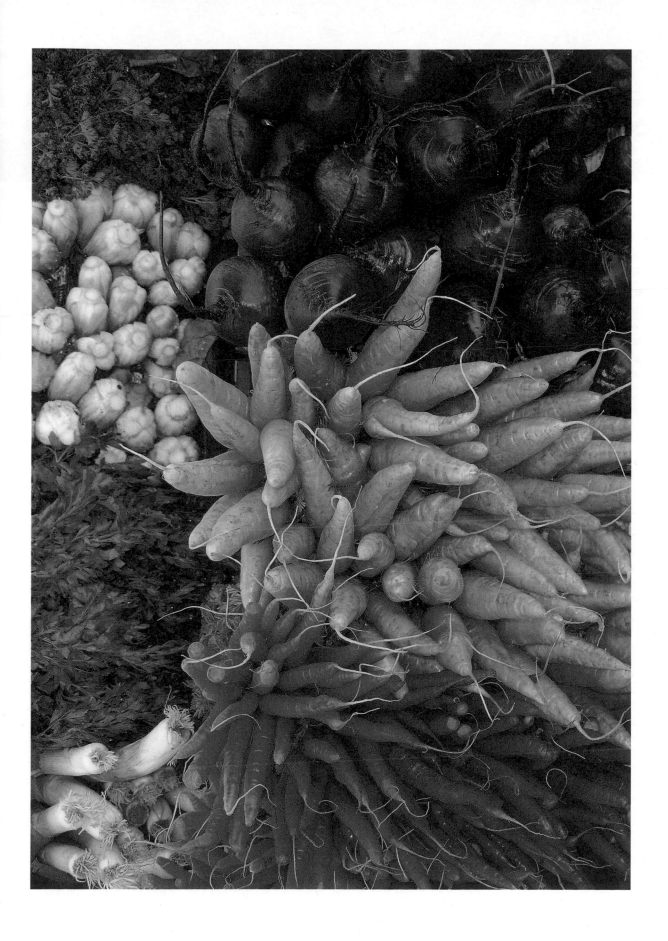

SAMPLE SESSION 1

So What About *Sow What?*

AT A GLANCE

Goal: Girls become aware of their place in the global food network as they start to think about where food really comes from and how their choices about food impact Planet Earth. They begin to customize their *Sow What?* journey in order to truly make a difference.

- **Opening Ceremony: Food Favorites**

- **The Real Food Network**

- **Food Prints**

- **Option: Flipping Your Food Miles**

- **Plan It: Food Forage**

- *Sow What?:* **Make It Your Own**

- **Closing Ceremony: Meal Memory or Attitudes of Gratitude**

MATERIALS

- **Food Prints:** large sheet of paper and markers or chalkboard; computer/ Internet access (optional)

- *Sow What?:* **Make It Your Own:** Photocopies of pages 42–43

- **Plan It: Food Forage:** Photocopies of pages 44–49

- **Flipping for Food Miles:** A few pieces of 8 1/2-by-11 paper or six 3-by-5-inch index cards for each girl; drawing materials; stapler

PREPARE AHEAD

Contact the girls in advance of the session and ask each to bring a favorite food, a label from it (if it has one), or a picture of it. No need to give detailed instructions. It will be fun to work with whatever turns up! Bring an item or two from your kitchen, too, if you can.

If it's not possible for girls to bring a food, ask them to write or doodle a favorite food on a slip of paper as they arrive at the gathering. Also photocopy the "Food Forage" sheets from pages 44–49, one set for each girl or each mini-team of girls.

Opening Ceremony: Food Favorites

Gather the team together and invite each girl to "present" her favorite food, explaining what she enjoys about it and where she usually gets it (homemade, from a store, etc.).

If the team has real food to enjoy together, now's a nice time to do that, too!

The Real Food Network

Now it's time for the girls to begin to envision all the resources—Earth's resources and people resources—as well as all the various decisions about those resources, that bring food to their tables. Invite girls to explore where their favorites they've named "come from" (besides the store!).

Start by asking: *How many people, animals, and resources of Earth—the sun, water, and air—go into getting our food to us?*

Ask the girls to choose a favorite food they've talked about today (or one ingredient in a food) and then tell the story of the web of interactions that brings that food to their table. They can make educated guesses or simply use their imaginations. But they must tell a whole story. You might say: *Start with what the sun did for it or what water did for it and move forward through all the steps that let this food reach its final destination—you!*

The girls might like to do this individually, in mini-teams, or as a large team. They can keep their examples simple—and have some fun, creatively capturing the story/web on a piece of paper or two. To get their stories going, ask them to consider questions like these that get them thinking through the a full "food time line":

Depending on the mood and energy of the girls and time available, they might like to add humor or drama by turning this into a guessing game or even a "mini-commercial" about their food favorites. If the team wants to get creative, they might enjoy spending a few minutes preparing to "perform."

Say your favorite food is an orange. Who planted the seed that became the orange tree? Who decided what kind of seed to plant and how? Where? Maybe in Florida? Who tended the tree? Was it treated with pesticides? Fertilizers? Artificial or natural? Who decided which kind? Where did that stuff come from? When the tree produced fruit, who picked it? Who tasted it? Packed it? Shipped it? Who unloaded it at the store? Priced it? Displayed it for you? Who bought it? How does it taste?

Invite each girl or team of girls to share her/their food network story. Then guide a short discussion:

- *How does our food connect us to Earth?*

- *How does our food connect us to people?*

- *When you bite into a piece of food, do you ever think about the people who produce it, pick it, or deliver it to you? Do you ever wonder whether they actually eat this food themselves?*

- *What are some of the decisions that are made along our food networks? How do they impact people and the planet?*

- *What ideas are we starting to have about how decisions along our food networks impact health—the health of the environment and our own?*

Encourage the girls to research, before the next gathering, more facts on their own to learn how close to the truth their network stories really come. Did they leave out any links in the web? Did they leave out any key people?

Food Prints

Set up a chart like the one at the top of the next page on a chalkboard or a big sheet of paper. A few examples are given in the chart, so either start the group with a blank chart or give them an example to get them started.

Then introduce this activity by saying something like: *Thinking about our food network helps us think about the impact our food choices have on the environment. Let's dig deeper! What is the "food print" of our favorite food?*

As the girls try to plot out where their foods come from, they may need to make some educated guesses for the moment. Encourage them to be curious! If they have access to the Internet (many teens can work wonders with their phones!), the girls might be able to gather some facts right now.

When the team has made a stab at charting out five or six ingredients, ask the girls to estimate the food print of each item, using this very simple rating: my state/region = 1; U.S. = 2; other country = 3.

Food	Ingredients	Where From Rating* *my state/region = 1; U.S. = 2; other country = 3
Tomato sauce on a pizza	Tomatoes Olive oil	Florida or Mexico (1, 2, or 3, depending on your location) California or Italy (1, 2, or 3)
Banana cream pie	Bananas Sugar Milk Flour	Costa Rica (1 or 3) Dominican Republic (1 or 3) 1 or 2 1 or 2
(a key local food from your region)		1

Point the girls to the COOL (Country of Origin Labeling) information on page 15 of their book, and also the mention of eatlowcarbon.org, the Web site that can help determine food miles. You might say: *These are good ways of estimating food miles, but for today's gathering, our simpler chart is just fine. The main idea to take in is that the farther food must travel to reach you, the greater the food miles involved and the bigger the food print it leaves behind.*

You might ask: *Anyone want to test that assumption? Making and testing assumptions is a big part of science, after all!*

Then say: *Now, let's step back and talk about it:*

- *What does the food print of our favorite foods tend to look like? Do our food prints vary, or do they tend to look similar?*

- *What kinds of items seem to have the highest food print?*

- *Do we have any items that scored a 1? Which?*

- *How much of what we are eating comes from our own region?*

- *Is that a lot or not much? If not much, could it be more?*

- *What could we be eating to be more local?*

- *What are the advantages to the environment of eating food from our region? Are there advantages to people and families in our region? Think about jobs and the economy. If we ate more locally, what would that mean for our community?*

- *Are there any advantages to us, too? (When does fresher taste better?)*

- *We just did a "quick assumption" about the food prints of our foods. What other factors contribute to the imprint our food choices leave on Earth?*

- *Should we consider how we carried it home from wherever we bought it?*

- *How much waste do our food choices create—food waste as well as packaging waste and utensil waste?*

Option: Flipping Your Food Miles

The girls might like to research more facts and create a "flip book" that shows and tells how their favorite food comes to their tables. They might even do this little by little, as the journey unfolds, and ultimately use their creation to educate and inspire others.

Pick a non-local fruit or vegetable and unearth as much as you can about how it reached your table. Break down what you learn into 10 to 20 scenes. Start the story as far back as you'd like, even with seeds or soil.

Then fold your paper into eighths (if using index cards, which are sturdier, fold them into thirds), and cut them apart. Draw one scene on each cut piece, leaving a margin on either the left or right side for a staple.

Staple your drawings together and start flipping. Use it to educate and inspire!

Plan It: Food Forage

A basic survival challenge that unites all people everywhere—across time and culture, and around the globe—is the need to find nourishing food.

Engage the Seniors in planning a small "food forage" event (kind of like a scavenger hunt) for your next gathering.

Hand out the "Food Forage " activity sheets from pages 44–49 of this guide.

Let the girls know the purpose:

- to explore the food print of the food available to us

- to find out what options we have

- to start thinking about how we can interact differently within our food network

- to have some fun with a "Team Twist" (see ideas on the activity sheets)

As girls check out the activity sheet, ask them what they might like to add, based on the ideas and conversation shared today. Also, what fun twists would they like to add to their outing? Note the ideas on the activity sheet and see if any are of interest.

Don't forget to ask:

* *While we are out "food foraging," what else might you like to do as a team for fun?*

* *Who can bring a camera or video camera? We might want to capture what we find.*

* *Are there any team challenges we want to add in—a little contest on who can find the freshest fruit, who has the funniest story to tell afterward, etc.?*

Encourage the girls to flip through their book for a few ideas they might want to keep in mind as they prepare to forage. Here are some places to start, and some suggested questions for the girls:

* The "Are You What You Eat?" section (starting on page 12) compares food miles for food grown locally and farther away.

* "Shopping the COOL Way" (page 15) describes "Country of Origin Labeling." Do any of the foods found on the forage carry labels like this? You might suggest that the girls check their kitchens at home and see what they find. They might also want to look for Fair Trade labels. Do they see any of these?

* "Mapping Your Pantry" (page 18) invites girls to plot out where their food comes from on a world map.

* "The Food Print of a Burger" on pages 16–17 is pretty interesting, too! What if you really did that?

* "From Variety to the Big 3" (page 47) describes how three crops— rice, corn, and wheat—make up 60 percent of the world's food. What do these monocultures mean for Earth? Now check the food favorites assembled by the group today. What are the rice, corn, or wheat components? What might they look for on your food forage?

* Page 44 is all about corn, which has a lot to do with, well, everything! For today, the girls might want to start by looking at how often "corn syrup" or other processed ingredients appear in their food labels. How is that "stuff" nourishing us? What does it do to our food prints? What labels might the girls check out on their forage?

FORAGE: WHERE AND WHEN? TOGETHER OR ON YOUR OWN?

Based on interest, transportation, and availability of adult helpers (you'll need more adults if girls want to divide into mini-teams and meet in different places), help the girls decide where and when they will conduct their "food forage."

Consider supermarkets, farmers' markets, food courts, restaurants, and small stores (bodegas, delis, convenience stores). Don't forget specialty stores like bakeries, and meat or fish markets, and food co-ops and health food stores.

If the team does not want to or can't gather for fieldwork as a team, offer girls the option of each exploring one or a few of the ideas on the "Food Forage" activity pages on their own.

You can then use a team gathering to share findings—and maybe even sample some foods together!

Sow What?: Make It Your Own

Here's a chance for girls to plan a *Sow What?* experience that really speaks to their interests! Present some of the options, following the ideas on the "Sow What: Make It Your Own" guide on pages 42–43. Encourage the girls to think about their preferences. They don't need to plan everything today. They can get some ideas going now and keep planning another all along the way.

Start by asking: *What interests you about the ideas in your book and the conversations we have been having today?*

If it's helpful, summarize the main point of this leadership experience. You might say something like:

> Sow What? *is a journey to connect with our food networks and the natural world and to create positive change that reflects a commitment to health, responsible decision-making, and a food network that's better for the environment!*

Invite the girls to discuss their interests related to each of these key food network issues (you may want to jot them down to help girls focus on them):

- The right everyone on Earth has to good, healthy, and affordable food.
- The importance of producing food through sustainable practices that protect Earth.
- Acceptable work conditions and fair pay for those who work on our farms, in our fields, and in our markets.

You might ask the girls for their ideas about how these issues interconnect with one another.

Let girls know that *Sow What?* will offer them many opportunities to get out and explore these issues—and also meet new people and talk to them:

> This Sow What? *journey is rooted in the real world, including farms, farmer's markets, supermarkets, restaurants, food banks, and more! We'll be going places and also bringing people in to talk to us.*

Encourage them to keep their interests in mind as they plan this journey experience—and, ultimately, their Harvest project.

Closing Ceremony: Meal Memory or Attitudes of Gratitude

Circle up and invite each girl to choose one of the following (try the other another time!):

- Briefly share the memory of a favorite meal and what made it special. Trying a new taste? Enjoying a familiar taste? The people who shared it? The time of year? The occasion? Laughter or ideas shared around the table? Ask one of the girls to capture key phrases about what makes a meal special on a piece of paper. Save it! You'll return to it in Session 3.

- Take a moment to express thanks for all of the resources—of Earth and people—that brought their favorite foods to them. They could do this with a moment of silence, by going around the circle and each saying one thing they are thankful for—without repeating each other—such as the sun, water, laborers who pick fruit, farmers who grow it).

- If the girls choose the second option, you might share this information about produce pickers on farms:

  Agricultural workers are among the most poorly paid workers in the United States. Tomato pickers, for example, often get paid 40–45 cents for each 32-pound bucket of tomatoes; they work 10–14 hour days, six days a week, and end up with an average yearly salary of $10,000. In Florida, the Coalition of Immokalee Workers (CIW) has spearheaded a human rights movement to improve wages and working conditions for farm workers. The CIW was able to negotiate one-cent-per-pound increases with Burger King, Taco Bell, and Whole Foods supermarket, which would increase the per-bucket wage from 45 cents to 77 cents.

You might ask: *After hearing this, how might you feel when you bite into a tomato, or eat tomato sauce?*

The issue of fair pay—for those who pick food, cook it, serve it, or clean up after it—may be a theme the girls want to explore throughout this journey.

You might also share with the girls the salsa recipes at right, which come from two CIW staff members, Nely Rodriguez and Silvia Perez. The Seniors might make a salsa to share at a future gathering, as a way of giving thanks to the workers who play such a key role in getting food to everyone's table.

SALSA CRUDA (RAW) OR COCIDA (COOKED)

- 4 ripe tomatoes, cut in quarters for raw salsa, left whole for cooked salsa

- 2 jalapeños, seeds, veins, and stems removed (wear rubber gloves when cutting hot peppers)

- ½ a handful of fresh cilantro

- ¼ of a small onion 1 clove of garlic (optional)

For raw salsa: Put all ingredients in a blender. If tomatoes aren't juicy, add a splash of water. Blend, then pour into a bowl and serve alongside tacos, tortillas, and beans, chips, eggs, meat—whatever you like.

For cooked salsa: Place whole tomatoes and trimmed jalapeños in a medium saucepan. Cover with water. Bring to a boil and cook for 10 minutes. Add the garlic, onion, and fresh cilantro. Place in a blender jar. Blend until smooth, but not liquid. Pour into a bowl and serve (as above).

Sow What? Make it Your Own!

THINK ABOUT . . .	WHAT WE'LL DO
THE HARVEST AWARD: Do you want to earn this prestigious Girl Scout leadership award? What do you hope to learn and explore by doing so? What interests do you have related to making your food network more environmentally friendly? Do you want to complete steps as individuals and discuss and share insights with the team? Or progress through the steps as a team? Will you use your gatherings primarily to work on the award, or mix in other opportunities along the way?	....
FREESTYLING: You might opt to "mix and match" ideas from *Sow What?* to create your own journey, and not focus on earning the award. What ideas from your book spark your interest? Perhaps you want to focus on exploring career ideas or use your energy on a particular topic covered in *Sow What?* There is no right or wrong way to journey through *Sow What?*	....
EXPLORING LOCAL FOOD: Yum! What would you like to spend time making and eating with your Senior friends? Cook off, anyone? Do you want to plan, prepare, and enjoy meals with guests, too? Ask your adult volunteer about the ideas offered in Sample Session 3. With a little imagination, you could create a whole journey out of them, or just plan some time to enjoy food along the way. You have plenty of recipes and other ideas in your book, too!	....
NETWORKING: Building a network of people will enrich your experience—and give you ideas and resources for college and career planning! Who would you like to meet along the journey? Agricultural experts or other scientists from a university? Business owners interested in sustainable food innovations? Restaurant and market owners? What do you want to find out by talking to them?	....

THINK ABOUT . . .	WHAT WE'LL DO
CEREMONIES: What (if anything) would you like to do to mark the opening and/or closing of your time together as special and apart from all the busyness of your daily life? Here are some ideas:	
• Would you enjoy sharing with your team both a good thing and a challenge you've experienced in life between Senior meetings?	
• Would you enjoy taking turns bringing in special foods to share?	
• What about rituals that various cultures use to celebrate food? (Check out pages 36–37 of your book to get you started.)	
• Would you like to practice a few minutes of quiet together, aided by a candle, music, or a beautiful photo of something in nature?	
• Take turns sharing poems, quotes, or music about nurturing yourself?	
• A blend of these ideas? None of these? Something of your own?	
How will your team share leadership? What skills and values will you offer?	
ADDITIONAL LEADERSHIP OPPORTUNITIES Perhaps you or other team members (or all of you in turn!) would like to lead the explorations and discussions at various gatherings. You could tailor and tweak and make them your own as you go). Find out which team members might like to "sign on" to lead. You can chat with your adult volunteer ahead of "your session" to get assistance in thinking the gathering through and adding your own creative touches.	
ENJOYING THE GREAT OUTDOORS How would you like to spend some time connecting to nature? Day hikes? A weekend camping retreat? Exploring places where food grows? Maybe you can link up with other Senior groups in your region who are journeying through *Sow What?* and have a mega campout with time to share ideas and networks, enjoying local foods along the way!	

TASTY NAME?

How about giving your team a name for this journey that represents food from your region? If you live in California, it could be the Santa Rosa Plum Circle; if you're in South Carolina, where the Provider Bush Bean grows, it could be the Provider's Council. Get creative! Get a little competition going with other Senior teams!

What's Available and What's Not

FOOD PLACES VISITED:

....

FRUITS AND VEGETABLES

What were the top three tasty-looking and ready-to-eat fruits or vegetables?

....

Why?

....

What labels did they have?

....

Where were they from?

....

What's their estimated food mileage or food print? Make a note about a few fruits for which you can calculate the food mileage or food prints.

....

What fruits or vegetables looked not so tasty/ready to eat?

....

Why not?

....

What labels did they have?

....

Did you find anything organic? Where was it from?

....

....

Did you find anything grown in this state? What?

....

WHAT IS MISSING?
Among the fresh foods you found, what was missing?

....

CORNY LABELS/PROCESSED FOOD
Read the labels on an assortment of packaged foods (cereals, cookies, chips). How many list "corn" as an ingredient?

....

How many list "corn syrup"?

....

How many list ingredients you're not sure of, or that don't sound like food? Make a note about a few ingredients you can look up online later.

....

NEAR AND FAR
Can you find any locally produced food? What?

....

What foods can you find that are made within 100 miles of your community?

....

What items seem to come from farthest away?

....

FAIR TRADE
Can you find any foods labeled Fair Trade? What? Where are they from? How much do they cost, compared to a similar product without a Fair Trade label?

....

....

COOL STUFF
What kinds of food items have COOL (Country of Origin Labeling)? Which don't?
What other questions could we ask about meat and dairy products?

....

Location	What's made there?	What's shipped in from other places?	Where do the key ingredients and supplies come from? (At the bakery, what grains are used?)	What's the most "locally made" item available?
SUPERMARKET				
FARMERS' MARKET				
FOOD CO-OP				
HEALTH FOOD STORE				
MEAT MARKET				
BAKERY				

Team Twists

TASTE, VALUE, FOOD PRINT: Everyone (or each mini-team) agrees to bring back the same item from a different place. Make it something that fits your budget and can be found in most stores. An in-season fruit, perhaps? When the team gets back together, compare notes on price, taste, label, and food print. Which came from nearest you? Farthest? If one was organic, can you notice a difference in taste? How about locally grown? Locally grown and organic?

ITEM	PRICE	TASTE	LABEL	FOOD PRINT

MAKING A MEAL OF IT: Agree on a simple, balanced meal with four or five ingredients—a protein, a carb, and a veggie or two. Perhaps chicken, a green vegetable, and a potato or rice dish. Price out these ingredients at various locations, and also a prepared meal that offers something as close as possible. Hint: Compare the "whole ingredients" of a dinner to fast-food and prepared frozen versions. What's the most economical option? Most convenient? Tastiest? Best for you and Earth?

OUR MEAL made from scratch:					Pre-Made Version (fast food or frozen)
INGREDIENTS					
COST					

VEGGIE TWIST: Do the above, but with a vegetarian meal. Make sure it includes protein and is something you would eat! Or have one team do a veggie twist and another do a "meaty" twist. Which one has the lowest food print? Which would you rather eat?

GO LOCAVORE: If you could only buy food grown and produced within 100 miles of your community, what would you come home with? Could you make a meal of it? What?

OUR LOCAL MEAL:				
INGREDIENTS				
COST				
CONCLUSIONS				

Talking It Up

Who can you talk to? Someone unpacking fruits in the produce aisle? The manager of the supermarket? A customer ahead of you in the line? The owner of a bakery? A cook at a restaurant? You can learn something new from all of them!

Here are some questions to get you started:

What is that you're unpacking? Do you recommend it?

....
....
....
....

What's the best value in your store this week? What do you recommend we try?

....
....
....
....

What leads you to shop at this store? How often do you go grocery shopping? Do you prefer shopping more frequently or less?

....
....
....
....

What's your favorite food to make from scratch?

....
....
....
....

Beyond the Food!

While out and about, keep in mind these topics. They influence the food network, and food prints!

Food advertisements: What words and images are used to influence your food purchases? What seems right? What seems wrong? What seems real? What seems fake? What do you wish you could find/see that you don't?

....

....

Convenience: Everyone's busy. Think about your family's schedule and lifestyle. How convenient is it for you and the adults in your life to shop at each place you visited?

....

....

Accessibility: Who could shop at each place you visited? Is there parking? Access by a bus or train? Could people bike (food print!)? How would people with disabilities shop there?

....

....

Customer friendliness: Is this a place you and your friends could go to? Why or why not? What if you shopped with food stamps? Had a very limited budget?

....

....

Role in the local economy: Who and how many people work here? Are people from your own community able to make a living here? What kind of living? Where do profits go? Who benefits? What charitable or community efforts does this business support?

....

....

Environmentally savvy: How much paper do you see being wasted? Plastic? Can you reuse your bag? Compost food? Recycle? How green is the building? What else do you notice about how much the habits here help or hinder the environment? How does all that add to a food print?!

....

SAMPLE SESSION 2
Foraging for Food!

AT A GLANCE

Goal: Girls explore the food network in their communities and gather ideas, information, and contacts they can use as they begin to think about changing some of the food prints they encounter!

- **Food Forage!**

- **Gather Up**

- **Plan It: What Makes a Meal Really Happy?**

MATERIALS

- **Food Forage!:** Copies of food forage activity sheets, pages 44–49; local map; camera or video camera for recording activities

PREPARE AHEAD

Based on the arrangements discussed at your last gathering, remind team members and adult helpers about where and when to meet.

Check in with your local Girl Scout council about any other safety advice relevant to your plans.

Identify a gathering place where the team can have a short chat about their findings and plan for their next gathering.

Food Forage!

Gather up and get to it! Remind everyone about staying safe—by sticking with designated team/mini-team and adult assistants, and not wandering off.

Encourage everyone who needs to exchange contact information to do so.

Make sure everyone knows where and when to gather back together to share experiences and make a few plans for the next gathering.

If the girls seem to need it, remind them about the purpose of this excursion:

- *We are checking out the food options in our community: What's available? And what's the food print it leaves on the environment?*

- *We are also going to try to talk to a few people along the way and see what we can learn from them!*

- *Have fun being out and about—think of it as a scavenger hunt!*

Gather Up

After the food forage, gather everyone together and capture the key ideas that are on the girls' minds. What pops for them? What is the most surprising, exciting, or difficult piece of information they've gleaned from the exercise? If you've done a "Team Twist," start there!

Here are some other questions to help guide the conversation:

- How much local food is available? How much is advertised?

- What evidence did you observe related to people (owners, workers, customers) trying to make decisions based on managing our food print/protecting the environment?

- What seems to matter the most to our community about food? Least?

- What does "food advertising" tell us?

- What is the impact of our food network on the environment?

IT'S NOT JUST THE FOOD!

As the team considers the challenge, think about the other environmentally friendly aspects of the gathering. Will you use (and discard!) paper and plastic plates and utensils? How about everyone bringing their own reusables? Compost bin? Transportation to and from? Carpool? You get the idea. How environmentally friendly can this gathering become? How about every Senior gathering? Now what is the food mileage and the food print?

WHAT'S FRESH RIGHT NOW?

The Web site of the Natural Resources Defense Council has a great way to find out what fruits and vegetables are in season in your area. You just type in the name of your state and the time of year and your receive the information, as well as recipes. Visit nrdc.org/health/foodmiles.

- How easy/hard would it be to make food shopping and eating decisions based on concerns for the environment? What would be easy? What would be hard?

- What ideas do you have about what is needed to improve our food network?

Take time, too, for girls to share funny stories and team moments of the day.

Plan It: What Makes a Meal Really Happy?

Ask the girls to decide how they'd like to conduct their next gathering, "What Makes a Meal Really Happy?" The goal is to spend time together enjoying a meal or snack that they prepare for themselves—one that is tasty and has the lowest food print possible! Besides exploring and enjoying food, what else do the girls want to do to make this a truly wonderful meal experience?

Consider these options (you and the girls may think of more):

- Depending on their time and resources, the girls might want to invite a few guests from the "food community." A food columnist from the local newspaper? A nutritionist? A farmer? A chef or entrepreneur? Someone with expertise in locally produced food?

- If the girls really want to go all out on a cooking and eating experience or event, turn it into a contest. They might want to add a gathering to the journey just for the planning. Otherwise, just choose one of the basic options below and you and the team can ramp up your e-mail and phone connections as you gear up for the next gathering.

- In mini-teams, girls each research and plan a recipe that can be made entirely (or mostly!) from products produced in the region. Depending on the season and what seems reasonable, set a distance range (50 miles? 100?). Their goal is to make a dish that they will enjoy sharing with the larger team—one that tastes good, feels good, and has low food mileage/a low food print (which they will track!). As an option, perhaps mini-teams want to compete: lowest food print, best taste? Who could judge? Would a local restaurant, store, newspaper, or even the school cafeteria feature the winning recipe?

- Do the above but as a whole team, either planning just one dish or snack or a whole meal to enjoy together. What's the food mileage and food print?

- Identify and enjoy a meal at a restaurant that features menu items made from scratch from local products. Talk to the chef or owner while you visit! What's the food mileage? The food print?

- If seasonably appropriate, just bring in "raw" items—fresh fruits, veggies, cheese, cider, bread—that are available locally and savor them together. If fruit is not in season and/or budgets are tight, jam from a regional maker (or homemade!) and bread will make a yummy option! Yes—think about the food miles and the food print!

DO IT UP IRON CHEF–STYLE!

Mimic the Iron Chef competitions of cable TV's Food Network! The girls can compete to create a dish from scratch—optimally, with a set and limited number of local foods, including one "mystery ingredient."

Some girls can be the producers, some the chef performers, some the hosts, and some the judges (unless the girls have invited outside judges). The producers will choose the ingredients for the competition. The performers will make the meals. The hosts provide lively commentary on the action. One girl should be the stage manager, and one should be a runner to help the judges.

Have the "chef performers" break into groups of two or three. Reveal the "mystery ingredient," and give each group some. Provide other ingredients and set aside no more than 20 minutes for the actual creation time.

When the food is ready, have the host talk to each group about their creations: What is it called? How did you prepare it? What is its nutritional value? How did you work as a team? Any issues you had to resolve in order to keep moving?

After the judges taste the creations, critique them, and select winners, the hosts invite the rest of the guests to taste.

HEALTHY RELATIONSHIPS COUNT, TOO

Let the girls know that as the team gathers together to enjoy the option they've chosen, they'll also have a chance to consider how relationships can either nourish them or sabotage them, just like food! Encourage them to consider what makes for healthy relationships in life and what gets in the way.

If any of the girls were a Cadette on the *aMAZE* leadership journey last year, have them dip back to think about some of the relationship strategies they learned there.

TOOLS AND PREP

It's a good idea to have most ingredients "prepped" ahead of time. But if the Seniors do need to use knives and other sharp utensils, be sure to have enough adult volunteers on hand to supervise so that the contest stays safe.

The girls might try to have some ingredients donated by a local farm or food purveyor.

WINNER FOR ALL

Perhaps the winning dish could be re-created and served at a school cafeteria. If so, the girls need to be sure to invite someone from the school food service to attend and judge. The other judges could be chefs, supermarket owners, farmers, farm workers, etc.

SAMPLE SESSION 3
What Makes a Meal Really Happy?

AT A GLANCE

Goal: Girls explore the pleasures of the "local harvest" as they explore all the "ingredients" that go into experiencing a truly happy meal. They compare this experience to some of their day-to-day encounters with food and the food network and then go on to think about what makes relationships nourishing, too.

- **Make It, Savor It!**
- **Dishing on Food**
- **So What Can You Commit To?**
- **Plan It: Dig Deeper**
- **Healthy Relationships at the Table and in Life**
- **Plan It: Sessions 4 & 5**

MATERIALS
- Whatever food and supplies girls need based on their plans
- Pen and slips of paper

PREPARE AHEAD
Based on the girls' ideas about how best to experience a "low food print" and fun and satisfying time together, remind them about what to bring and other logisitics for this gathering. Has anyone identified and invited some guests they could learn from? Maybe you know some? And remember, any time girls are interacting with adults from the community is a good time to encourage them to ask questions that will give them new insights into career and educational possibilities, too!

WHAT'S A LOCAVORE?
A locavore is someone who eats food that has been grown locally, rather than food that may have traveled by truck for many miles. The term was coined in 2005 by four women—Jen Maiser, Jessica Prentice, DeDe Sampson, and Sage Van Wing—in San Francisco. The idea is to eat only food grown within a 100-mile radius of where you live. *Locavore* was named the word of year by the *New Oxford American Dictionary* in 2007.

Make It, Savor It!

Engage the team in preparing and enjoying the meal/snack/dish they have planned. In addition to the food, what else do girls want to put into the occasion? Music? Candles? Poems or quotes about food? A themed conversation about . . . ? If you have guests, invite them to share what they know, and encourage the girls to ask questions.

Encourage the girls to calculate the food print, and the overall footprint, of the experience. Has it changed since the first gathering? How? Chat a little about what the impact would be if more people were more aware more of the time about their food decisions.

Dishing on Food

As the experience of enjoying the food winds down, engage the team in a discussion about what truly makes a meal a happy experience. Below are some ideas to use in the discussion. No need to use them all! You might even like to start with the sheet of ideas girls put together during the closing ceremony at your first gathering.

- *Fresh ingredients vs. processed foods with lots of stuff you're not sure really is food. What's the difference in your mind? In your body?*

- *Do you feel good knowing you ate something made from "good stuff"?*

- *How does it feel to actually take time to think about what you eat, find the ingredients, put a meal together, and sit and enjoy it? How is this different from what you often do?*

- *What was the food print of this food? How does it help or hinder Earth's food network?*

- *What from our gathering besides the "food print" has left a mark on Earth? What can be done about that?*

- *Whom do we have to thank for the ingredients of this meal? How does our consumption of it help or hurt them?*

- *Besides the food itself, what else can make enjoying food a wonderful experience? People? Sharing ideas? Taking time away from "busyness"?*

COACH TOWARD A GREAT TEAM EXPERIENCE BY:

- Complimenting the ways in which you see girls working together, balancing talents and interests, etc.

- Asking girls how they feel about their teamwork. What do they feel great about in their interactions with each other? What would they like to work on?

So, What Can You Commit To?

Now encourage the girls to use what they have been discussing to choose a personal habit they can change—because it will help Earth (and them, too). What gets in the way of them truly nurturing themselves? Does this hurt Earth, too? What promise would they like to make as they attempt to replace this old habit with a new one? Encourage the girls to concentrate on one specific habit—no need to overhaul their whole lives! Success is more likely that way. You might suggest this activity:

> *If you eat processed snack foods every day at a certain time (bags of chips or cookies), maybe you'd like to make a new ritual for yourself instead. Jot it in your journey book, or on a slip of paper you will carry, or in your journal. When you write it down, do so from a positive place. Don't use words like "don't," "won't," "stop." Here are some more ideas:*

- *When I get home, I will enjoy 15 minutes of playing my favorite peaceful song while I wash and cut fresh fruit and eat it from my favorite plate.*

- *On Tuesdays, I'll buy my favorite bread from the bakery and enjoy it by . . .*

- *Once a week, I will organize my family to sit down and talk together while we are eating.*

- *I'll organize friends to go with me to the farmers' market or _____ twice a month.*

Maybe the commitment is even something girls want to do together, as a team, when they gather. For example, how could the team reduce its food print and footprint at their gatherings? How can they work together as a team?

Once girls have made their commitments, ask them if they want to share them with one another. Would they like to buddy up for support? Would they like to take a little time at upcoming gatherings to check in with one another?

Also, take a moment to ask the girls to think about the impact that personal promises can have on the Earth's food network. How will they calculate their reduced food prints?

Healthy Relationships at the Table and in Life

While girls are preparing the food and eating together, get a discussion going about how much more enjoyable it is to share food among people who have healthy relationships. Here are some questions to guide the conversation:

- *Who do you most enjoy sharing meals with?*

- *What do you talk about while you eat?*

- *What do you consider a healthy relationship?*

- *What kinds of behaviors do people show in healthy relationships?*

- *What kinds of conversations happen or don't happen in unhealthy relationships? (Backstabbing? Gossip? What else?)*

- *What happens when you share a meal with people you have unhealthy relationships with?*

- *What's one strategy you want to commit to in order to have more healthy relationships in your life?*

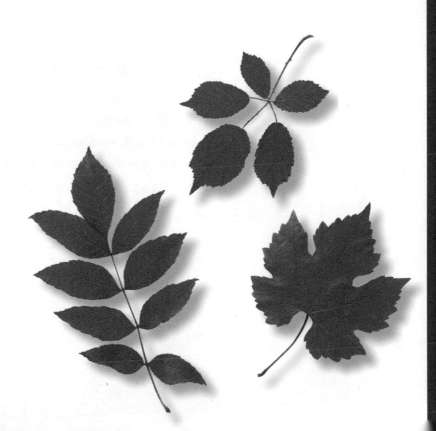

Plan It: Sessions 4 & 5

Take time to engage girls in planning the upcoming sessions. Perhaps they even want to divide into two groups: Dig Deeper (agricultural practices) and Sow What: Global Outlook (global hunger).

Take a few moments to plan for a team opportunity to "enjoy some dirt" on food by learning more about the agriculture or science behind food in your region. Depending on time and resources, this would be a great opportunity to also think about how the team can get outside and enjoy nature together. Maybe the outing could even involve a visit to a university. Offer these ideas about where the team could go and whom they could talk to:

- A farm (or search for a representative from the local chapter of Future Farmers of America)
- A farmers' market
- State department of agriculture
- University department of agriculture

If none of these seem feasible, consider:

- Connecting with a volunteer from a community garden or an avid gardener or two who grow veggies in their yard or window boxes.
- Finding a mycologist or a savvy food forager—fresh wild blueberries, anyone?—and ask for a guided hike.

Encourage girls to start thinking about what they'd like to learn and ask! Perhaps they can peek ahead at the "Dig Deeper" questions offered in Session 4 and see what interests them or what they'd add.

PLAN NOW FOR SESSION 5, TOO!

Share with the girls the options for exploring issues of world hunger on pages 66–69 of your guide. Which one do they want to chose? Or perhaps they want to do several and spend more time on this, possibly even adding in another session. Encourage them to get in mini-teams and plan it out, including drawing up a list of materials or guests they'll want to invite.

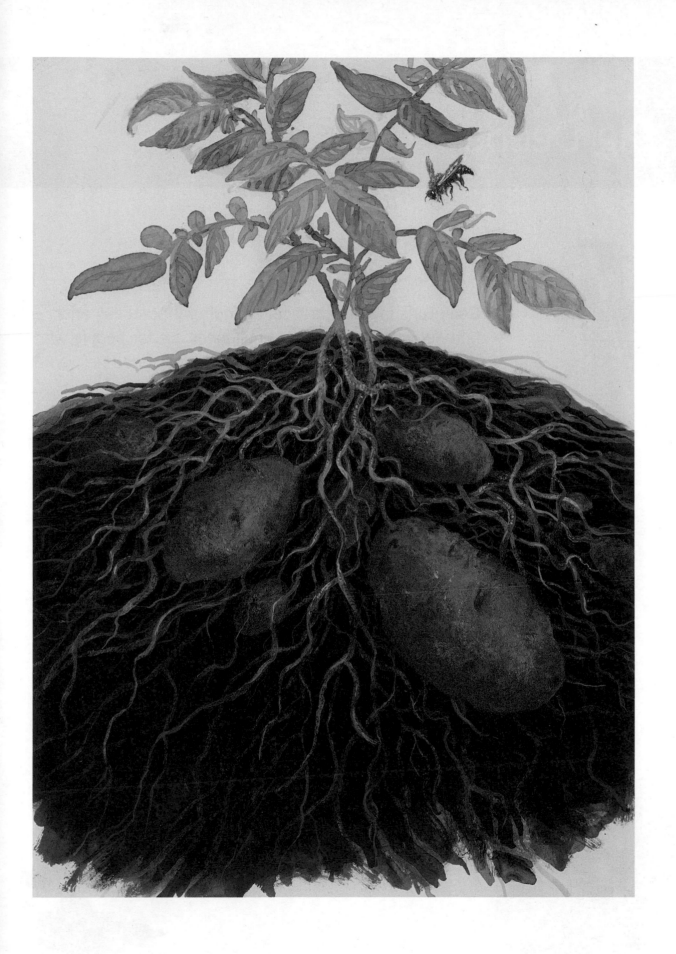

Dig Deeper

AT A GLANCE

Goal: Girls investigate local agricultural practices and find out what some of the challenges are for people who produce food in their region for the larger food network.

• **Dig Deeper, Get Curious!**

MATERIALS

• **Dig Deeper:** Whatever materials the girls need for their investigations and chosen options

PREPARE AHEAD

Based on interest, time, and resources, talk with the girls and adult helpers to finalize logistics for this gathering on digging into the agricultural and scientific side of food.

Depending on where you are going and whom you are talking to, encourage the girls to bring a soil sample (see page 29 of their book).

Dig Deeper, Get Curious!

As the girls are out and about talking to people involved in growing food in their region, use the handout of questions on the following page to get them thinking.

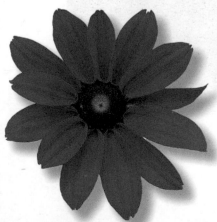

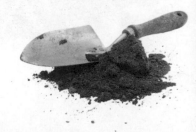

Dig Deeper, Get Curious!

As you're out and about talking to people involved in growing food in their region, keep the conversation going with these questions:

What do you grow/produce? Why?

....

Who are your customers? (Or who uses what you grow/produce?)

....

What challenges do you face? What can be done to ease them?

....

How do you produce your product?

....

Do you use artificial fertilizers? Other techniques?

....

What technology do you use?

....

Has new technology enabled you to do anything differently? (Has it changed? Does it yield improvements? Do you shun technology?)

....

Who and what do you learn from? What did you need to learn to do this work?

....

What did you study? Any learning by doing?

....

Where does the stuff you produce start from?

....

Where does it end up?

....

Where are you in the food network?

....

More Time, More Interest?

Depending upon the logistics of your gathering, here are some other things the team might find interesting:

Five Fun Things to Do Along the Journey with Friends: The activities featured on "wood frames" on this page and the next offer some fun and uplifting ideas (they're also featured on pages 10–11 of the girls' book).

All in the Family: What present or past food growers/producers/locavores are in your own family history—in this country or in a whole other part of the world? Find out! Share!

Away with Waste: One way to eliminate food waste and to play a role in weaving together loose ends left over in our modern food system is to create a compost pile or bin. Composting is a way of recycling food scraps and other household and backyard organic matter, by allowing them the time and space to decompose, after which they can be returned to the soil. There are various methods for composting. Where you live—in an apartment or house, or on a farm—will determine the style that's best for you. If the girls are interested in composting, consider contacting a master gardener through a state agricultural extension office.

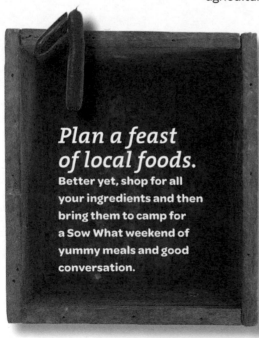

Plan a feast of local foods.
Better yet, shop for all your ingredients and then bring them to camp for a Sow What weekend of yummy meals and good conversation.

Talk about your values.
Sound corny? When do you really get to express who you are and what you stand for? Share what you value, hear what your friends value. Then, in a sisterly way, help one another live up to these values. (Check out all the women profiled along this journey. What are their values? How do they live them? Which of their values match your values?)

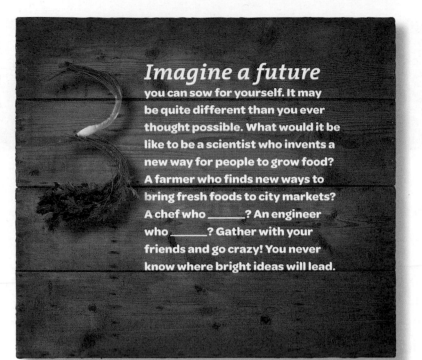

Imagine a future

you can sow for yourself. It may be quite different than you ever thought possible. What would it be like to be a scientist who invents a new way for people to grow food? A farmer who finds new ways to bring fresh foods to city markets? A chef who _____? An engineer who _____? Gather with your friends and go crazy! You never know where bright ideas will lead.

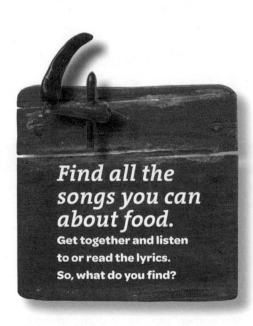

Find all the songs you can about food.

Get together and listen to or read the lyrics. So, what do you find?

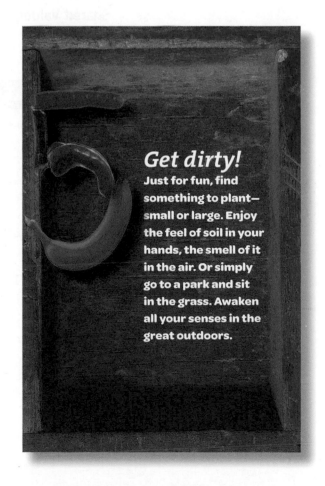

Get dirty!

Just for fun, find something to plant— small or large. Enjoy the feel of soil in your hands, the smell of it in the air. Or simply go to a park and sit in the grass. Awaken all your senses in the great outdoors.

SAMPLE SESSION 5
Sow What?: Global Outlook

AT A GLANCE

Goal: Girls consider the values represented by the various women featured in their books, and how they and these women are connected. They then focus their attention on the global issue of hunger, considering how their own decisions and actions impact the food network around the world.

- **Opening Ceremony: Shared Values**
- **Hunger Pain**
- **Closing Ceremony: Gratitude**
- **Plan It: Toward the Harvest**

MATERIALS

- **Opening Ceremony: Shared Values:** Slips of paper photocopied from page 71 (or your own versions on recycled paper)
- **Hunger Pain:** Whatever materials or foods the girls need for their chosen option

PREPARE AHEAD

Copy and cut up the names of the women and girls featured in the girls' book, from page 71 of this guide, for use in the Opening Ceremony.

Opening Ceremony: Shared Values

Put the names in a bowl or bag and invite the girls (individually or in mini-teams) to choose one. Give everyone a few minutes to read about the person they drew in their *Sow What?* book, focusing on these guiding questions (which you might want to jot down on a large sheet of paper or board):

- *What is one value that this woman/organization is focused on that I also value? How does the person/organization live this value?*

- *How do I live this value?*

- *How is this value represented in the Girl Scout Law?*

- *How does trying to live this value connect girls and women around the world?*

- *How does trying to live this value make this person and me leaders?*

Gather the girls in a circle and invite them to take turns expressing their insights about the values they share—with the Girl Scout Law and with women around the world.

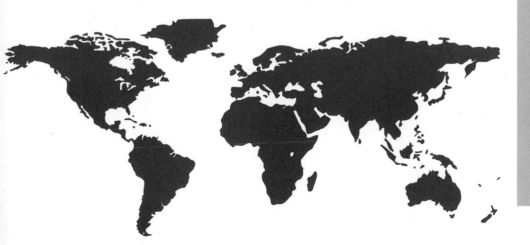

TURN UP THE MUSIC!

There are many songs from around the world that express ideas about working the land and cultivating food. Encourage girls to explore some and bring them to a gathering to share. Play them in the background of the Hunger Pain discussion, too! What do the lyrics have in common? What are some timeless human themes about sowing the Earth?

CONNECT THE DOTS

Encourage the girls to try the "Mapping Your Pantry" exercise on page 18 of their book, which asks them to open their kitchen cabinets at home or go into a food store and check out the label on single-ingredient goods. How do their food maps look? Do they tend to differ or are they all the same? What does this tell them about their food networks?

OPTION: FOCUSING ON FOOD WORKERS

Remind the girls of the tomato workers in Florida that they learned about in their Closing Ceremony for Session 1 and how they joined together to secure better wages. (If the girls didn't make use of that information on page 41 of this guide, share it now.)

Remind the girls that it is possible to be a key member of the global food network and yet not be able to afford to eat well. Some workers may not even be able to afford to eat the foods they pick or serve!

What workers might they locate in their region to discuss these issues? Once they understand the issues, what might they do to improve the situation? Is this something that they can pursue for their Harvest Award project?

Hunger Pain

Based on the plans the girls began in Session 3, guide them as they put one or a blend of the options in motion to explore why the global food network does not feed everyone and what could be done about it.

No matter what option the team is using, here are some suggestions for starting the conversation and harnessing their best insights on the topic. Encourage the girls to add their own insights and questions!

- *Who decides who gets to eat what? How do public policy decisions impact people's food choices?*
- *What decisions get made—about agriculture and other issues—that contribute to hunger?*
- *How does poverty impact the food choices people make?*
- *What decisions can be made that would help to solve hunger?*
- *We've all heard/felt the notion "You can't mail your excess/leftovers" to someone who is starving, yet intuitively we can feel that "excess here" must have some impact "there." What are your ideas about this?*
- *How does hunger impact the choices people can make in life?*
- *How can science contribute to solving hunger? What can't science do?*
- *What does the "status quo" do for hunger around the world?*
- *Why is hunger often described as a woman's issue? How do you feel about that?*
- *What innovations are happening around the world that could help?*
- *What would you advocate to change?*

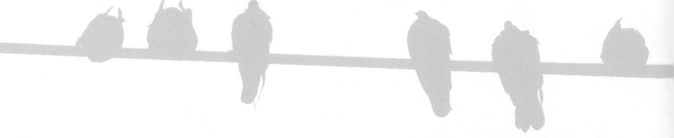

OPTION A: GLOBAL PERSPECTIVES

Identify one (or a few!) guest speakers who can visit the group to talk about their firsthand experiences with global hunger.

- The Seniors might consider former members of the Peace Corps. Contact the organization's Speakers Match at peacecorps.gov/wws/speakersmatch/ or e-mail info@peacecorps.gov to invite returned Peace Corps volunteers.

- Staff or volunteers from a local refugee resettlement agency or an organization involved in providing support to immigrants.

- Members of the religious community or armed forces who have perhaps served in an impoverished country.

- Staff or workers from international relief organizations, such as CARE, Oxfam International, Save the Children, or Heifer International (check for a chapter, committee, or office located in your region).

- Agricultural experts or other scientists working to improve food-supply conditions. (Try your state university extension services.)

- Health-care professionals: doctors, nurses, nutritionists, or other health-care providers who have worked with hunger victims.

OPTION B: HUNGER'S LOCAL, TOO

Identify people involved in combating hunger in your area: those who run food pantries, emergency shelters, food stamp programs, or school breakfast and lunch programs.

WHERE YOU ARE, WHAT YOU SPEND

In some parts of the world, and some parts of individual countries, people are able to spend less to eat high-quality, fresh food.

What can the girls learn about the differences in food spending right in their own region? How do neighborhood food prices vary? What differences do they see? What neighborhoods have low prices? Which have higher prices? Does this seem logical or illogical? Why?

What might the girls do to even out the situation? Could this be a Harvest Project worth pursuing?

OPTION C: EAT FROM ANOTHER PERSON'S PLATE

Divide your team into three groups. Get three scraps of paper. On one, write "$25 per person." On the second, write "$7 per person." On the third, "$1 per person."

Mix up the slips and have each team pick one.

Now, plan a meal based on the "money" your team "received."

Depending on your team's time and resources, you can either go all out and actually prepare a real meal or just create it on paper, based on food advertisements and menus in your area.

Once the "meals" are ready, bring the three teams back together and compare the food. Which group has the most? Which the least? Which meal would you most prefer to eat? Why?

You and your team did this as a learning exercise. But think about how this scenario and far more extreme ones play out as an everyday reality at meal times around the world.

How would it feel to eat the $1 meal when people at the next table are (possibly) eating the $25 meal? How would it feel to eat the $25 meal when others nearby are eating only $7 or $1 worth of food? Which meal would you want to eat each day? Why?

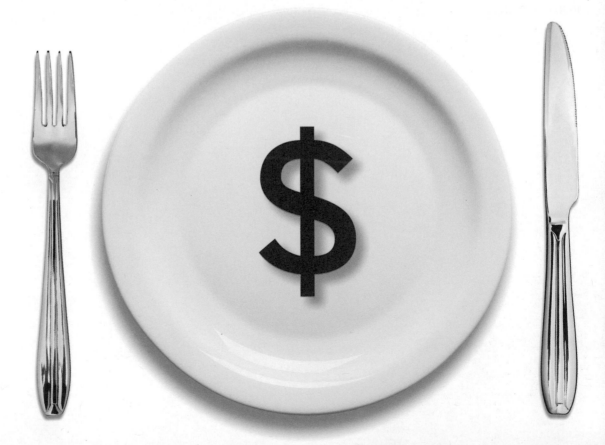

OPTION D: USE THE MEDIA

Opportunities for girls to network directly with people are best, but if that's not possible, the team could explore the issue of hunger via photographs, documentaries, articles (in print or on the Web), and videos, such as those available at wfp.org/videos, part of the Web site of the World Food Programme, the United Nation's frontline agency in the fight against global hunger.

The Peace Corps site, peacecorps.gov/wws/multimedia/videos/index.cfm, also has videos that can be downloaded:

- "The Last Drop" (peacecorps.gov/wws/multimedia/videos/lastdrop/) explores Jordan's water situation through interviews with national and local officials, water researchers, and average Jordanian people. The video was filmed by a crew of Jordanian girls and Peace Corps Volunteer Susan Miller-Coulter.

- In "The Growing Challenge in Senegal" (peacecorps.gov/wws/multimedia/videos/senegalsoil/), filmed by returned Peace Corps volunteer Clare Major, former Peace Corps volunteers Cory Owens and Clare Major show how they worked alongside farmers in Senegal to improve their crop yield and help them organize.

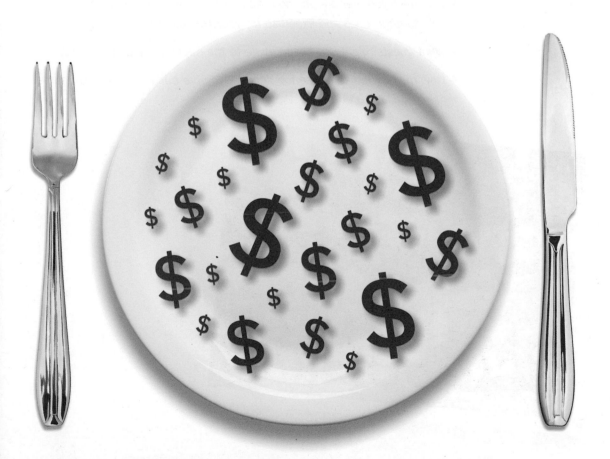

Closing Ceremony: Gratitude

Exploring the pain caused by hunger around the world can stir up a lot of emotions. Before wrapping up this gathering, perhaps the girls would like to spend a little time sharing their own gratitude for the food and nurturing they have in their own lives.

They might have their own way to do this—a song, poem, grace, or other ritual they enjoy with their families that they would like to share with one another. Remind the girls to be respectful of the various ways they and their families might choose to express gratitude. Alternatively, girls might like to create their own gratitude ceremony on the spot—which could be as simple as creating a team gratitude collage, by each writing or drawing on a shared piece of paper.

Plan It: Toward the Harvest

Let the team know that at their next gathering, they will think about a Harvest project they would like to pursue, either as individuals, mini-teams, or one large team. The goal of the project is to contribute positively to the food networks they have now explored in the world around them. You might ask:

- *What would you like to do to get your creative juices going ahead of our next gathering?*

- *Who have you met and learned from so far on this journey who might be able to offer ideas and expertise for your Harvest project?*

- *What guests might you like to invite to the upcoming planning session?*

- *How might you like to use the network you are building to also get some career advice?*

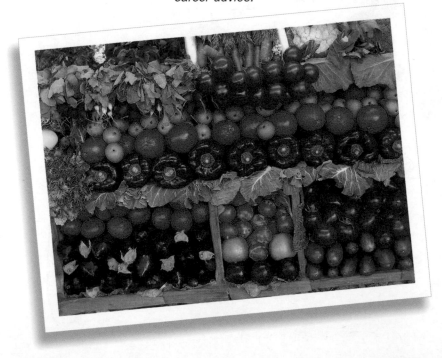

SHARED VALUES

COPY AND CUT ALONG DASHED LINES.

STACY LEVY
The Food Web as Visual Art

SHARI ROSE
Getting Kids to Eat Their Veggies

BARBARA EISWERTH
No Fruit Tree Left Behind

SIV LIE
Cooking with and for People

LYDIA SOMERS AND IVY VANCE
Restoring Iowa Prairies

MOLLY MORRISON
Listening to the Land

SUZANNE STRYK
Sharing an Awe for Nature

JUDITH REDMOND
Pest Control Without Chemicals

LADONNA REDMOND
Caring for Community

MARY CATHERINE MUNIZ
Recipes That Work

MIRIAM MANION
City Farms, City Food

KAREN BLAINE
Reconnecting with Culture

DENISE O'BRIEN
An Oasis of Biodiversity in a Sea of Corn and Soy

ANDREIA BORGES
Making the Most of the Land

SARAH SCHWENNESEN
Raising Corn-Free Cows

Planning to Harvest

AT A GLANCE

Goal: Girls identify their project for the Harvest Award. They also check in on their teamwork and discuss the importance of speaking up in healthy relationships.

- **Opening Ceremony: Seeds of Wisdom**

- **Commitment**

- **Teamwork and Healthy Relationships**

- **What Will We Harvest?**

- **Advocacy and Policy**

- **So, What About the Law?**

- **Closing Ceremony: Planting Hope**

MATERIALS

- **What Will We Harvest?**: Photocopies of the Harvest Planner on pages 80–81 for the girls (or their own version made on recycled scrap paper)

PREPARE AHEAD

Assist girls in selecting some of the community members they have been meeting and cultivating along the journey to come to the gathering and help them shape their Harvest project. If they can't attend, maybe they can share some ideas beforehand or help with implementing the project. Adjust the ideas provided in this session based on the expertise and ideas of any guests who will join the gathering.

Use the Harvest Plan pages (78–79) to stay on top of all the ins and outs of the girls' Harvest project. And give the girls their own planner, which you can photocopy from pages 80–81.

Opening Ceremony: Seeds of Wisdom

Start by saying something like: *Since we began our* Sow What? *journey, we have explored our food network from many perspectives. Let's each share one new "Seed of Wisdom" we are thinking about as a result of something we learned or experienced.*

(If girls have been enjoying capturing their ideas on a "team collage," they might like to do so again now, each adding a seed of wisdom to a team expression).

Commitment

Take a moment to check in with the girls about how they are doing and feeling about the "commitment" they made to themselves during your earlier gathering. Does anyone want to share progress? Get support for a struggle? Change their promise? Add a new one?

It's important to also ask girls what they are learning about themselves—and the food network—just by trying to keep their promise!

Teamwork and Healthy Relationships

Take time to check in on how the girls are doing with their teamwork, and with their relationships—with their Senior friends and in wider circles of life.

You might ask: *How do you speak up in a team? How do you speak up in a healthy relationship? What's similar? What's different?*

Get the girls thinking about relationship conversations with a simple scenario, such as: *Your friend wants to X. You would really rather Y.* (Ask girls for examples.) Then get a dialogue going with questions like: *What do you say? Are there times when you're afraid to speak up? Why? What holds you back? Have you ever spoken up and regretted it? Why? When do gossip and backstabbing get in the way of healthy relating?*

Then ask: *What communication do you expect to give and get in a nourishing relationship? Do you find that you usually get what you are wanting?*

Conclude by having girls talk a little about how they are doing as a team in preparation for undertaking their Harvest project.

What Will We Harvest?

Start by letting girls know that the Harvest project is an opportunity to strive toward making a lasting change in the food network around them. Lasting change comes from thoughtful planning and action, aimed at some root causes of issues, and includes a plan for the effort to keep going. The effects of their project should last beyond the time and resources that the girls themselves put into it.

Engage the team in a discussion:

- *Why is effort toward ongoing change important?*
- *What happens after "one-shot" events?*
- *What are some examples of change efforts that are actually quite simple but get at the root of an issue and continue on—or spread?*

Remind the team that with good planning, a change effort might not take a lot of time and resources, but could still lead to meaningful results. Ask: *Can anyone think of an example?*

Now, start the brainstorm for a Harvest project! Perhaps girls want to volunteer to guide the discussion, write down ideas, etc. Do they have their own thoughts about running the brainstorm and coming to a decision? Will they vote? Discuss until a consensus develops? Other thoughts?

Share with the girls the "Guiding Principles for a Successful Harvest" on page 77. What would they like to add? If you have guest experts available, encourage them to contribute ideas, too! Let them know that as they develop an idea, they will use this list to check that they are headed in the right direction! As needed, get the ideas hopping with these suggestions:

- *Check out the ideas offered on pages 90–93 of your book.*
- *Look at the "seeds of wisdom" ideas shared today. What projects might they lead to?*
- *What have we learned from some of the people we met? What project ideas have they suggested?*
- *What ideas from the personal "Promise?" efforts you are engaged in could benefit more people?*

MORE FOOD FUN

With all this planning going on, if the girls are looking for a fun food "do," check back on the options for Session 3 (What Makes a Meal Really Happy?) and do one the group hasn't yet tried.

Also, look ahead to Sessions 7 & 8 for activities about careers, monoculture, and sewing.

- *What does your food network ask of you? Or, what can you persuade other people to learn and do for the food network?*

After an assortment of ideas have emerged, encourage girls to check the ideas using the "Successful Harvest" list. You might ask:

- *What ideas best stack up to the list?*

- *Should any ideas just be crossed off?*

- *How will the group come to a final decision?*

Once the team has an idea, they can work out a specific plan for achieving it.

Advocacy and Policy

Get the girls thinking about what it means to advocate for policy change. Advocating means speaking up to influence decisions and get the resources and support needed. Here's an example to share: *Say you are interested in starting a school vegetable garden. You would most likely first need to speak up to get the land and resources and support needed to plant the garden. You might speak to the principal, the school board, the PTA—or all of these and more! You'll have to find out who can influence which decisions and then speak up for the decisions that will aid your vision. That's being an advocate. As you can see, influencing in this way is necessary before anyone can begin to prepare the soil or plant any seeds!*

Be sure to talk to the girls about how their Harvest project doesn't need to "do it all." What can they advocate for that gets change going? Who can they connect with so that the change can continue and grow?

Also, remind the girls: *Putting a plan in place to advocate is important, even if a decision-maker ultimately says no. This project is about trying and learning to keep trying.*

You might also let girls know that in the future, as Girl Scout Ambassadors, they can try the leadership journey *Your Voice, Your World!* and walk through all the steps of being an advocate.

IF THE TEAM IS STUCK . . .

. . . maybe they just need more time to decide on their Harvest project! Would everyone like to think about the project and come back at the next gathering to decide on it? Or maybe they need some more examples and insights? Who else can they talk to or visit to come up with better ideas?

So, What About the Law?

Now that the girls have a plan in the works, encourage them to read the Girl Scout Law on the inside back cover of their book. Ask:

- *Which lines of the Law will your project help you live?*
- *Which lines will it educate and inspire others to live, too?*

Closing Ceremony: Planting Hope

For any project to be successful, the organizers have to be full of hope for the impact! Invite girls to gather in a circle and have them share their hopes. Ask:

- *What do you hope your project will accomplish?*
- *How do you hope to learn and grow from this project? As a team?*
- *What kind of snowball might you start with your project?*
- *How, ultimately, will this help Earth or demonstrate your love for Earth?*

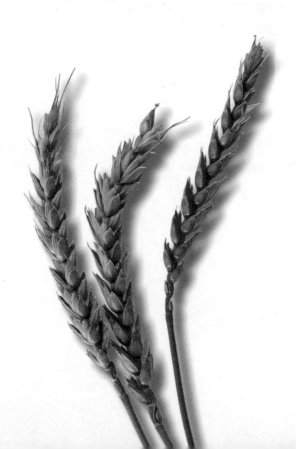

Guiding Principles for a Successful Harvest

Encourage the girls to review the guiding principles of a great Harvest project on page 88 of their book, and share with them this expanded version:

A successful Harvest project:

- Helps the girls expand their network—they get to meet and interact with some new people!

- Gives team members a chance to use talents and skills in new ways. The girls will all face a challenge—one they are excited about. (Speaking out, persuading others, doing good for Planet Earth!)

- Identifies a specific problem and involves the girls in a specific solution—not so big and broad that they can't do it and feel the impact.

- Is doable with the time and resources the girls have. For example, they may want to try to incorporate it into their school day.

- Gives girls a chance to practice advocating—speaking up to try influencing a policy or resource decision (asking for land to be used for a garden, requesting that a restaurant serve local foods).

- Gives girls an opportunity to educate and inspire others to be involved, too.

- Strives for a sustainable impact, no matter what its focus. The girls may push for a new policy or for a change in an existing one. They don't need to start something from scratch.

And don't forget to emphasize for the girls a key theme of this journey:

- Everything they do for their Harvest project represents their care for Planet Earth and all of its inhabitants! As the theme of this journey makes clear: It's Your Planet—Love It!

HARVEST PLANNER

Our issue:

....
....
....

Our goal:

....
....
....
....

What we will do (and where and when):

....
....
....
....
....
....
....

Why this matters and how it will benefit the planet and people:

....
....
....

HARVEST PLANNER

Experts in the team's network that we will tap	Area of expertise	Contact info

HARVEST PLANNER

Project tasks	Who does it?	When due?

HARVEST PLANNER

We'll educate and inspire people by . . .

Along the way, we'll make time to . . .

We'll be a great team because . . .

Harvest Time!

AT A GLANCE

Goal: Girls team up and carry out their efforts to have a positive impact on the food network, en route to earning their Harvest Awards.

Depending on the time the girls have and the nature of their project, they might be doing their Harvest project for one, two, or more sessions. Use the coaching tips here to guide them.

The specific activities you and the girls choose for these sessions will depend on their interest and their Harvest project. A variety of activities are offered here that the girls might enjoy apart from, and along with, their project.

- **Harvest Project Coaching Tips**
- **Impact Circle**
- **So, What If . . . Career Possibilities**
- **Monoculture, Anyone?**
- **Relate S'More**
- **Create a Food Ceremony or Festival**

MATERIALS

- **So, What If . . . :** Depending on the team's interests, some basic art supplies such as markers, glitter, glue, magazines to cut up, paper, unused sides of old poster boards, file folders, etc.

- **Monoculture, Anyone?:** Music, a way to play it, or varieties of one food (see page 88)

PREPARE AHEAD

Use the Harvest Project Coaching Tips to assist you in guiding girls on their projects, and engage the girls in the other suggested activities as time allows.

Copy or write the career roles listed on page 87 on slips of paper and put them in a jar or bag. If the girls want to go artistic with this activity, ask them to bring in the desired art supplies.

Ask girls to bring in examples of music they really like, and ask a volunteer to supply electronic equipment to play it on. Optionally, the team can also bring as many varieties of one kind of food as they can find (apples, potatoes, etc.).

HARVEST PROJECT COACHING TIPS

No matter what kind of project the girls are doing, keep in mind that it's not just "what" they do, but how they go about it and what they learn through trying that will inspire them to take action throughout their lives! These coaching tips will help you keep the team on track.

❏ WHO CAN YOU MEET?

It's important for girls to expand their networks. New people = new ideas + new opportunities. If they are creating an advertising campaign on behalf of a farmers' market, can they talk with professionals who work in advertising? Perhaps they are asking their school to designate land for a garden. Who can assist them in planning their presentation? What could they learn from talking to a school board member? You get the idea—the more people girls meet, the more authentic and purposeful their projects will be! Ask girls and their families who they know and who those people know. You don't need to know everyone yourself.

❏ CONSIDER THE POWER OF MORE

As in, what are other Girl Scouts, especially Seniors, doing in your region? Maybe other girls on a *Sow What?* journey have similar interests. How can girls benefit by teaming up with more peers? How can their projects benefit?

❏ KEEP IT REALISTIC

It's great for girls to have big ideas—the world needs them! Just gently remind the girls to keep their current effort focused around the time and resources they have available. They will have more success that way. And success might lead them to do more!

❏ MEET A TRUE NEED

Maybe girls think their community needs a vegetable garden and they start a plan to organize one. With a little investigation, they might find that there are already several community gardens—and what is really needed are more volunteers to keep the gardens going. They could focus their time on recruiting volunteers instead. Regardless of their interest, a little investigation will ensure that girls' efforts are spent on an area where they can make a difference.

HARVEST PROJECT COACHING TIPS

❏ TRY FOR SUSTAINABILITY

Using the above example, go one step further. Let's say girls find that a community garden needs volunteers and they decide to volunteer for a day or two. Then what? Alternatively, if they use their creativity to recruit other volunteers, they will have an impact long after earning their Harvest Award!

❏ SUPPORT GIRL ADVOCACY EFFORTS

Speaking up is an important way to "do good." Give girls plenty of encouragement and practice! Someone needs to present the plan to town officials or the school board, or ask for a policy change. Guide the girls to speak for themselves. And reward their courage. There may be times when adults don't take them seriously. They may not even return their phone messages or e-mails. At that point, you might step in to initiate a meeting or call and then hand it back to the girls.

❏ TALK ABOUT IT!

Yes—we all like to do, do, do. But taking key moments to talk about what they're doing is an important part of the girls' learning experience. What is hard? Why? What does it take to work around a challenge? What will you miss if you give up? If a plan is not working, how can you adjust it? What is fun about this project? What are you proud of?

❏ TEAM DYNAMICS

Take every chance that comes up to give the girls positive feedback about their efforts as a team and to coach the team through bumps. When a conflict arises, you can say something like: *I notice you seem frustrated with one another. Let's talk out all sides and see the problem from each perspective. Then we can try to solve it!* When things are going well, offer observations like: *I love how you really use and rely on one another's skills to solve problems together.*

❏ SHARE!

Girls can use what they learn and do to educate and inspire others! This is an important way for girls to build confidence and realize that what they do really does matter. Sharing their project is a great way to also strive toward sustainability . . . maybe others will be inspired to act, too! Girls can share their efforts in big or small ways, using their creative juices. How could younger girls benefit? Maybe a family meeting with parents? A presentation at school or a place of worship? Online networking? The possibilities are endless, and girls can choose the way that suits their time and interest. Even "small" efforts deserve to be shared!

Impact Circle

Here's a simple example of how you can engage the girls in a meaningful moment or two to recognize the impact their project can have in the world:

Call the team into a circle and invite each girl to offer her response to one of these statements:

- *Our project is important because . . .*
- *I am proud of our effort because . . .*
- *Our project helps the food network by . . .*

The girls might jot their responses on a team collage or a piece of scrap paper. They might like to return to these ideas as they wrap up their journey.

So, What If . . . Career Possibilities

The many interesting women featured throughout *Sow What?* have chosen career paths that the girls might not ordinarily think about. By now, the Seniors have also met some new adults in their own food networking (growers, scientists, retailers, chefs, and entrepreneurs).

Here's a creative exercise to engage the girls in using these connections to think about what is possible for their futures: Take out the jar or bag holding the slips of paper with the career roles listed on page 87. Then invite the girls (in pairs or individually) to choose a slip of paper.

Now ask each girl or pair to try on the role they drew—just for today (no one needs to make a commitment!). Here's the extra challenge: They need to think about—and describe—how they would use their role to benefit the food network (and the people who rely on it). Some girls might groan a bit and "hate" the role they drew. Encourage them to give it a try, just for fun. They might gain new insight into themselves!

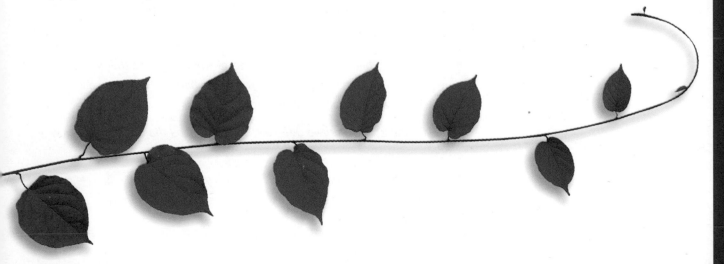

Give the girls time to put together a story about what their life could be like if they had this role. Then have the girls share their stories with one another. Depending on time and interest, girls might like to draw or diagram or create some other fun way to show what it might be like. Perhaps act out a scene? If girls want, once they have gone through one round, they can return their roles and pick new ones.

Here are a few prompts for anyone who needs a little boost to get started with her story:

- *What would you need to learn? What would be interesting to you about that? What would be hard? What would you do to learn this information?*

- *Where would you live to do this kind of work?*

- *Whom would you love to meet and work with?*

- *How would you use your role to have a positive impact on Earth? What specifically would you try to do? What benefit would your work have?*

- *What challenges would you face in doing this work? Would you face any additional challenges as a woman doing this work? How would you handle them?*

- *What kind of equipment would you need?*

- *What shoes would you wear? What food prints and leadership prints would you leave behind?*

- *How long could you see yourself in this career?*

AFTER EACH GIRL PRESENTS . . .

Once all the girls have had a chance to try on a role or two, huddle up and discuss what girls have learned by thinking about these varied career possibilities. Here are some questions to get the conversation going:

- *What is different about the kind of careers you thought about today from other ideas you have had in the past? What's the same?*

- *How do people figure out career directions?*

- *Do you think there could be some kind of work out there that you don't even know about that might make you really happy? How can you investigate and be open to many possibilities?*

- *Do you think women have different career options than men? Why or why not?*

- *What "ingredients" would be part of a job you would really like—e.g., opportunities to meet lots of people? To be creative? To make a difference?*

If I was a farmer I would

If I was an agricultural researcher I would

If I was a restaurant owner I would

If I was a chef I would

If I was a store owner I would

If I was an artist I would

If I was an inventor I would

If I was an advertising executive I would

If I worked at a school I would

If I was a nutritionist I would

If I owned an import/export company I would

If I was a coffee-bean taster and buyer I would

If I was a _____ I would

If I worked for an international relief organization (Peace Corps, Red Cross, CARE, etc.) I would

ONE FOOD, MANY VARIETIES

If your time and meeting place allow, try as many varieties of one kind of food as you can. Sliced apples are a simple choice. If you can boil water, try different varieties of potatoes (perhaps with a pinch of salt, pepper, and butter). Talk about the different choices. Do girls have different preferences? Why or why not? Do they enjoy having the choices?

Monoculture, Anyone?

Ask the girls to check out pages 47–51 of *Sow What?* Ask: *Why do you think biodiversity is important for the food network and the people who rely on it?*

If the girls have brought in music, say: *Name a song, musical artist, or group that you like a lot. Play that music if you've got the equipment! Take turns. Think about the music you listen to at different times of the day and week and when you are in different moods. What are all the different influences wrapped up in this music? Make a list. Not sure? Guess a little.*

(Alternately, if the girls brought in varieties of a food, have them share and taste!)

Then say:

- *Look at your list. What if there were only one kind of music in your world? What would you miss?*

- *Now make some lists of your "top 5" or "top 10" outfits. What about movies, television channels, or radio stations you enjoy? Restaurants? Celebrities? Foods?*

- *Check out your various lists. What kinds of differences do you enjoy? Why? What do you learn from these differences?*

- *How about on teams? What kinds of different strengths, skills, ideas, and qualities make up a great team?*

- *Think about this—could we describe some parts of our lives as a "monoculture?" Consider: the people you sit with at lunch or hang out with during free time? Your friends? Girl Scouts?*

- *How do monocultures come about in our lives? Do we plan it that way? What might we be missing when we spend our time in monocultures? Is there anything we might like to think about changing?*

Relate S'More

Engage the girls in a conversation about how they are doing on their healthy relationship efforts started back in Session 3. You might ask:

- *Who has tried a new relationship strategy? What was it? How did it work out?*

- *What gets in the way of good relationships? How does backstabbing and gossip hurt? How can you protect yourself from it and how can you not do it yourself?*

- *Thinking back on "monocultures," what's great about having relationships with all different kinds of people—in terms of gender, culture, ethnicity, geographic, physical ability? How does it add to your life?*

- *What are the different beliefs that people you know have about relationships?*

- *How do girls relate to one another? How do boys relate to one another?*

- *Do girls and boys relate differently with one another?*

- *Wrap up by writing your "recipe" for a great, healthy relationship. What tips do you recommend? What do you advise staying away from? You might even want to use your recipe to educate and inspire younger girls.*

Create a Food Ceremony or Festival

Check out pages 36–37 of *Sow What?* for ideas about how societies around the world honor food. Ask the girls what ideas they like. Encourage them to trade ideas about how their families honor food.

Also take note of "Fun with Food Festivals" and "New Ritual for a New Day" on page 39. Get inspired and, as a team or in mini teams, create a special way to honor a food you enjoy. Your idea can be simple or complex. You can map out the idea just for fun or you can plan it and do it!

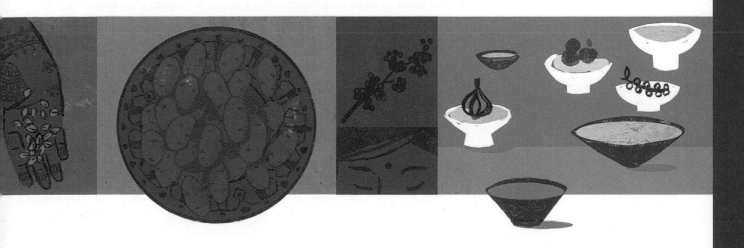

Reap What You Sow!

AT A GLANCE

Goal: Girls conclude their *Sow What?* journey, assessing what they have learned, connecting with all those who have assisted them, and celebrating their Harvest.

- **Harvest Time! (Seeds of Fun, Seeds of Inspiration, Seeds of Ceremonies, Seeds of Thanks, Seeds of the Future)**

MATERIALS

- **Harvest Time:** Photocopies of the Harvest Time! pages for girls (91-95) and whatever the girls need for celebrating the journey and their accomplishments

PREPARE AHEAD

This sample session offers a "bountiful harvest" of ideas. The girls on your team might want one, two, or more gatherings to use them! Consider these suggestions as possible starting points to guide the Seniors to create their own fruitful ending to their journey, with opportunities to:

- Take pride in what they have learned about the prints they leave on Earth—leader prints, food prints, and maybe even . . . ?

- Thank all those whom they have met along the journey for sharing time and insights.

- Share their Harvest projects with others and see if any ideas emerge about keeping the effort going.

- Celebrate among themselves and with whomever else they might like to include.

Harvest Time!

Seeds of Fun

S'MORES WITH A TWIST

A warm, toasted marshmallow oozes into chocolate, and two graham crackers sandwich the sweets together. What's the food print of all that? How about a S'More-Off? In mini-teams, invent a new kind of S'More. Whose recipe has the lowest food print? Whose uses Fair Trade ingredients? Who used the lowest food miles to acquire the ingredients? Get imaginative! Who can judge?

MORE MEALS—REALLY HAPPY!

If you liked the ideas your adult volunteer provided for Session 2 and want to do one again or try a new one, now's the time—just ask to review them again! Have you tried any of the recipes in your *Sow What?* book? How about inventing one of your own?

Our *Sow What?* Recipe Ideas:

....

....

....

....

MYSTERY MEAL PARTY

Do like Siv Lie on pages 30–31 of your book. Each girl on the team can bring an ingredient. So, what will you make?

....

GET OUTSIDE

If you have not yet had a *Sow What?* outing, don't miss an opportunity to camp, hike, or enjoy a day at the park together. Talk about what you most love about Earth! Sun, air, water, soil! Trees, flowers, animals and . . . So much to love, so much to take for granted—unless you get out a little and enjoy! Check out page 54 in your book, where Molly Morrison is profiled. Find a land trust near you!

I'd like to visit:

....

....

SOW WHAT ELSE? (AND MAYBE EVEN SEW!)

Of course, crops that grow on Earth don't just produce the food we eat. They produce lots of other stuff we use, like cotton for clothing, sheets, blankets, and so much more! What's the story of some of the cotton lying around in your home? An old shirt from your mom? A summer dress from when you were younger? A worn-out comforter?

Gather some fabric scraps or just one item and find an imaginative way to tell the story. Who grew the cotton? Where? What soil, air, sun, and water made it grow? Who made it into what it became? How did it get to you? What's a happy memory about how you or your family used it? If you are in a crafty mood, think about how you can creatively use the scraps to tell the story. Mini quilt? Senior team quilt? Fabric collage? What else?

I'd like to make:

....

....

Seeds of Inspiration

What have you learned and experienced that you want to share with others? How will you do that? How can you reach out further to leave your leader print on Earth?

FOOD PRINTS

Now that you know about your food print, who else in your life can you inspire to think differently about how they participate in the food network? What is one habit you could inspire lots of friends and family members to change? Start simple. Where could the snowball go? What activity can you get people to try—to give them a *Sow What?* moment of their own?

....

....

How could you use your imagination to get some younger Girl Scouts to start thinking about their food prints? Would a flip book help (ask your adult volunteer for the details, given in Sample Session 1 of her journey guide)? Could you post your call to action on the Internet? In a newsletter at your place of worship? In the town newspaper? Make a display for the library?

....

....

LEADER PRINTS

What have you learned about who a leader is? Does a leader have to be the person at the front pulling everyone along? What do you do that makes you a leader? What kind of leadership do you think Earth needs? Make a commitment to providing some of it! Then share it with others (Younger girls? Your family? Friends at school? A teacher or two? Who?) and ask them to make a leadership commitment, too!

....

....

Seeds for Ceremonies

Maybe you and your sister Seniors have earned your Harvest Awards. Maybe not. Either way, take a little time to capture what you've learned and share it with one another. Ceremonies can be a great way to highlight the important moments of your journey experience. Here are a few ideas to get you started (add your own creative sparks!):

Gift One Another: Tell one another (or write a note, even in your books) about the personal values and talents that you admire. Make it serious (I admire how you speak up about what you believe; I love your curious questions—they help me learn). Or make it fun (You get the award for team jokester, most hip, most neat and tidy). Even make it symbolic (I gift you with a little packet of sunflower seeds because you always make get togethers feel bright and sunny!).

Name It: Say one thing you learned on your *Sow What?* journey—something about yourself, your food networks, leadership, or a little of each! Capture it on paper, in a jar, or in a collage. Pass on your wisdom. Share it with Girl Scout Cadettes. Encourage them to keep the wisdom growing!

Commit to Your Leader Print: Promise to look out for more opportunities to be a leader in your world. Think about how you'd fill in the following statements. Then share your ideas with friends.

I was pleased to Discover that a value that is important to me is ....

I will keep living this value by ....

When I Connect with other people in the community, I ....

I will make more connections by ....

I think it is important to Take Action to ....

In the future, I'd like to Take Action to ....

Put Your Heart In It: *Sow What?* is part of the *It's Your Planet—Love It!* series of leadership journeys. Why do you love Earth? What does the planet do for you? What will you do for it?

Seeds of Thanks

Who are all the people you have talked to and learned from along the way? How will you let them know what gifts they have given to you and how much their interest and time has meant to you? From people you talked to on your food forage to the farmers or scientists you spoke to as you were digging deep, from everyone who did something to move your Harvest project along to the adults who drove you around—don't leave anyone out of your network of thanks.

Your thanks can range from simple and heartfelt notes, to sharing a tasty (and low-food print!) treat, or a photo or drawing that represents an idea you learned with someone's help. What other ideas do you have about giving thanks? As you use your creativity to show your gratitude, remember that people networks, just like food networks, need your care and attention. Whom have you met who can help you with school, or with ideas about college or careers, or maybe even reference letters? Keep your new network thriving. Thanks is a good way to start! And, of course, don't forget to sow some gratitude for the Girl Scout volunteers who have guided you along the way.

Seeds of the Future

Before you end your *Sow What?* journey, be sure to investigate other opportunities in Girl Scouting that might interest you. Check out *destinations* at girlscouts.org and think about taking a trip—across the country or around the world! When's the Cookie Activity Program? You might be able to earn some dough for travel. What are other teen Girl Scouts up to in your area? Ask your council for an event list or check online.

So, what will you find? You won't know until you ask!

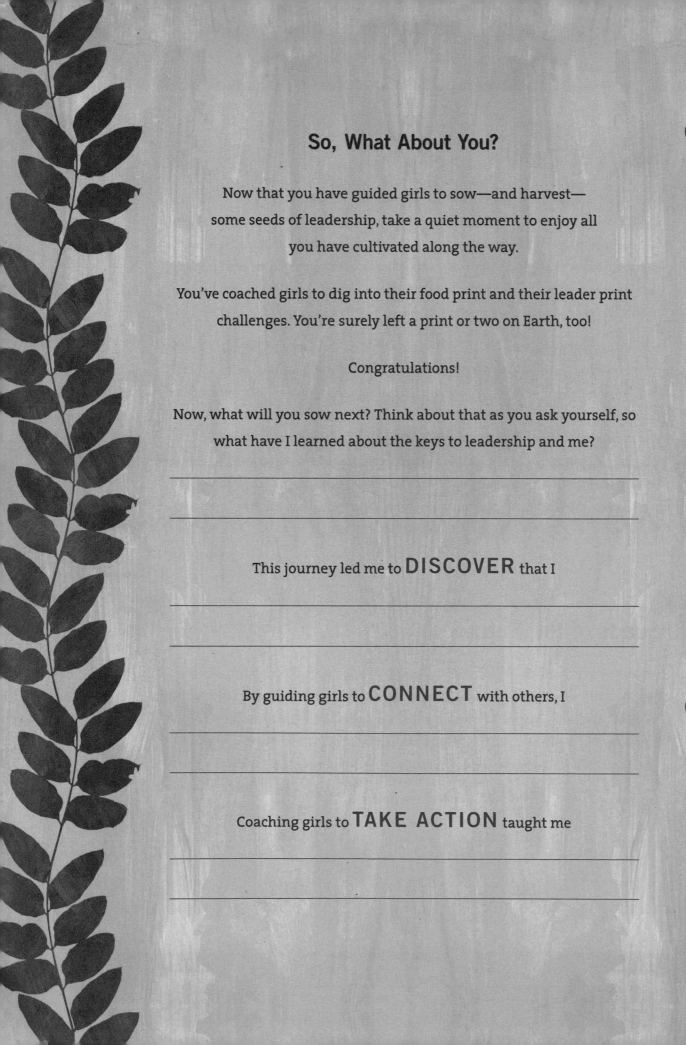

So, What About You?

Now that you have guided girls to sow—and harvest—
some seeds of leadership, take a quiet moment to enjoy all
you have cultivated along the way.

You've coached girls to dig into their food print and their leader print
challenges. You're surely left a print or two on Earth, too!

Congratulations!

Now, what will you sow next? Think about that as you ask yourself, so
what have I learned about the keys to leadership and me?

_____

_____

This journey led me to **DISCOVER** that I

_____

_____

By guiding girls to **CONNECT** with others, I

_____

_____

Coaching girls to **TAKE ACTION** taught me

_____

_____